Mystic Healers
&
Medicine Shows

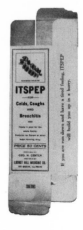

Mystic Healers

&

Medicine Shows

Blazing Trails to Wellness
in the Old West and Beyond

EDITED BY GENE FOWLER

Ancient City Press

Santa Fe, New Mexico

Book design by John Cole
Cover illustration by Faith DeLong

International Standard Book Number
0-941270-94-7 clothbound
0-941270-95-5 paperback

Library of Congress Cataloging-in-Publication Data

Mystic healers and medicine shows: blazing trails to wellness in the
    Old West and beyond / edited by Gene Fowler.
        p. cm.
    Includes bibliographical references (p.).
    ISBN 0-941270-94-7 (cloth:alk. paper). —ISBN 0-941270-95-5
(pbk.:alk. paper)
    1. Healers—West (U.S.)—Biography.
    2. Medicine—West (U.S.)—History.
    3. Quacks and quackery—West (U.S.)—History.
    4. Medicine shows—West (U.S.)
    5. Frontier and pioneer life—West (U.S.) I.Fowler, Gene, 1950–
R153.M97 1997
615.8'56'097—dc20   96-34432
                                                      CIP

10 9 8 7 6 5 4 3 2 1

Disclaimer

Mystic Healers and Medicine Shows was written to convey a lively account of folk healers
and spiritualists on the American frontier from the 1870s to 1930s. It is not in any way
intended to be used as an herbal medicine book. The formulas are given here solely for
their historical value.

Contents

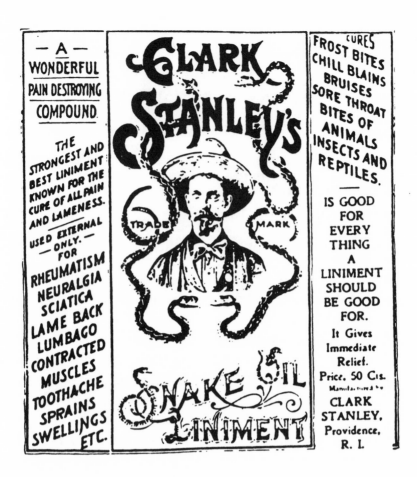

Advertisement for Clark Stanley's Snake Oil Liniment, circa 1890s.
Courtesy Center for American History, University of Texas at Austin.

Introduction
Sawbones, Spirits, and Snake Oil

GENE FOWLER

Has it ever seemed odd to you that people are so fascinated with outlaws of the Old West? That Billy the Kid has become a sort of James-Dean-on-the-frontier sex symbol? That we seem transfixed by endless reenactments on stage, page, and screen of psychotic desperadoes plugging fellow citizens with hot lead?

We're a bit obsessed with the shoot-em-ups, all right, but what about the patch-em-ups? Somebody had to deal with all that famous carnage. Poor old Doc on TV's "Gunsmoke," for instance—every time his mustache dipped into a cold beer he'd get called from the saloon to dig a slug out of Matt Dillon or some scoundrel the marshal shot down on the street. With all the bloodletting on the frontier as depicted by pop culture historians, it almost seems a miracle anyone survived to settle the West.

The story of pioneer and frontier medical practitioners has not been completely neglected, of course. Richard Dunlop chronicled trailblazing medicos such as Dr. George Goodfellow of Tombstone, Arizona, in *Doctors of the American Frontier*. The trigger-happy populace of the "town too tough to die" provided surgeon Goodfellow with a laboratory for surgical research in the 1880s. In *Southern California Practitioner* and other medical journals, Dr. Goodfellow published articles such as "Cases of Gunshot Wound of the Abdomen Treated by Operation" and "Note on the Impenetrability of Silk to Bullets." Though his medical skills were apparently state-of-the-art for the time, Dr. Goodfellow penned some creative autopsy reports. A bandit hung by a Tombstone mob died from "emphysema of the lungs, which might have been and probably was, caused by strangulation, self-inflicted or otherwise, as in accordance with the medical evidence." Examining a dead gambler, Dr.

Goodfellow "found the body to be rich in lead but not too badly punctured to hold whiskey."

Dunlop also captured the story of California's Dr. Thomas D. Hodges, aka stagecoach-robbing "Tom Bell." When the doc's second job landed him in prison in 1855, he used his medical knowledge to feign illness, then escaped from the prison hospital. Once when a gang member shot a stagecoach occupant reluctant to hand over valuables, the robber-doc dug out the bullet. Then he bandaged the victim, paid a passing wagon driver $10 to haul the injured man to town, and rode off with the rest of the loot.

Robert Karolevitz tracked the medical side of westward migration and settlement in *Doctors of the Old West: A Pictorial History of Medicine on the Frontier.* One full-page photograph captures the startling white mane of Dr. John McLoughlin. Often called the "White Headed Eagle," McLoughlin performed medical and administrative duties for the Hudson Bay Company in the Pacific Northwest, earning a second title, "the Father of Oregon."

Karolevitz's caption for a photograph of Dr. Brewster M. Higley says that the heavily-bearded physician "traveled westward to Kansas to rebuild his life after a losing battle with demon rum and a broken marriage. On the secluded banks of West Beaver Creek in Smith County, Doctor Higley built a tiny cabin" and penned a poem that would become the lyrics of a classic western folk song, "Home on the Range."

Both works point out that, prior to World War I or so, "regular," or allopathic, physicians trained in the era's mainstream medicine were often outnumbered by "alternative" practitioners—folk curers, herbalists, faith healers, homeopaths, "rubbing doctors," patent medicine promoters, and medicine shows.

This book, *Mystic Healers and Medicine Shows*, profiles a dozen or so assorted medical mavericks, along with one or two colorful "regulars" shuffled in as wild cards. The time and place of their medical practices range from the 1870s to the 1930s and from the Wild West to the Midwest.

Many of these frontier-style healers took advantage of the western tradition that encouraged self-invention. Some intentionally created a new persona, even going so far as to rename themselves after noted frontier figures such as Kit Carson and Big Foot Wallace, or at least to take on a suitably exotic appellation such as Arizona Pete or Apache

Jack. For others, the transformation seems to have been made by a force of nature that was unavoidable. In either case, their distinctive self-images went hand in hand with their singular and innovative treatment methods.

Like other frontier folk, due to the dearth of doctors, early Californians welcomed any kind of practitioner. One of the earliest doctors in Los Angeles, John Marsh, arrived in 1836 when the City of Angels was a pueblo of 1,200 people. Delighted when Marsh produced a Harvard diploma, community leaders endorsed his practice. The only problem was, the diploma's Latin text stated that Marsh had not graduated from Harvard's School of Medicine but from its School of Letters.

Many became healers based on local need. Nancy "Grandma" Parker arrived in West Texas in the early 1870s and soon became her area's unofficial doctor. She first settled in a dugout near Tokeen (later called Content) and then moved into a one-room log cabin. There she brewed medicinal teas and tonics in a huge pot, using herbs gathered from the wild country around her. Grandma Parker found the redroot plant effective for diarrhea and broomwood tea good for coughs, while the bitter balmony weed was a lift for biliousness. She treated asthmatic children with candy made from the mullein plant, and she also gave the herb to asthmatic adults, who received relief by smoking it. Her cabin still stands about sixteen miles northeast of Winters.

Many pioneer German-Russian communities in the Plains states received health care from healers, generally female, who practiced an Old World "supernatural folk medicine" known as *Brauche*. This "magico-religious healing," as folklorist Don Yoder defined it in "Folk Medicine," uses "words, charms, amulets, and physical manipulations in the attempt to heal the ills of [human] and beast." Anthropologist Timothy J. Kloberdanz collected information on about seventy such healers, including Salomea Dockter, who settled with her family in North Dakota in 1889, where she soon gave birth to her thirteenth child in a wagon box. "Eventually," writes Kloberdanz, "the Dockters' isolated homestead became familiar to hundreds of travelers, including expectant mothers and persons seeking health care."

The remote Big Bend country of Texas utilized the services of numerous informal physicians. J. O. Langford, a thirty-one-year-old Mississippian, moved his family to Boquillas Hot Springs on the Rio Grande in 1909 and soon cured himself of malaria with the hot mineral water. Word spread, and Langford became a hydropathic medicine man. (On occasion, however, this process worked in reverse. Dr. Henry Hoyt arrived at Fort Elliot in the Texas Panhandle in the 1870s, where sick folks were so scarce the physician had to find work as a cowboy.)

William Money, renegade California physician, theologian, astrologer, and historian—described by William B. Rice in *William Money: A Southern California Savant* as Los Angeles's "outstanding eccentric" of the nineteenth century—arrived in about 1840. In the next fifteen years, he reportedly treated five thousand patients with only four casualties. "Perhaps," wrote Rice, this record was achieved "through the dosage of such remedies" as those the settlers had added to Indian nostrums. "Sulphur, lard, raw potatoes, roasted cactus leaves, and freshly killed chickens were used in poultices. Nursing bottles might be made of cow horns fitted with buckskin nipples. To cure a toothache the California physician might have ordered his patient to carry in his mouth the eye-tooth of a man or a black dog. For pleurisy the victim often drank a potion brewed from fresh horse manure."

Impromptu communities that sprang up around northern California goldfields after 1849 also hosted imaginative health-care providers. George Groh described several in *Gold Fever*. One such "picaresque figure" at Placerville was a Dr. Hullings, "a tall, heavy-bodied man who swaggered about in a costume of blackcoat, Mexican sash, and velvet *calzoneras* of bright green. He was said to be competent enough when sober, but his usual condition was drunk." A "vicious brawler," he was rumored to be on the lam from a New Orleans killing and brutishly drove off others who dared hang a shingle at Placerville.

One who earned Hullings's wrath was the university-trained Dr. Edward Willis, who killed the hard-drinking Hullings in a duel. Willis's pine board-and-sailcloth tent/office provided a marked contrast to the usual gold camp clinic. "There was a microscope," wrote Groh, "a stethoscope, a glittering array of surgical instruments, a mortar and pestle, some chemical retorts and alembics, an assortment of medications and splints, and a great jar of leeches." Several anatomical specimens were preserved in alcohol, but "just for show," the physician explained to a friend, "because the miners expect them." It seems most folks anticipated some kind of entertainment with their medicine.

Viewed a century or more later, there is an inevitable aspect of the dramatic to most every element of life on the western frontier. And an air of magic and mystery surrounds the healing arts in any age and place, often marking the physician as an extraordinary being with uncommon powers. That is certainly true of the unique medical personalities profiled in this book.

Some of them brandished theatricality with a flourish. The Diamond King's fifty-cent and one-dollar bottles of Spanish Oil may or may not have cured consumers, but odds are his show lifted folks' spirits enough to help their bodies mend. There were hundreds of similar troupes crossing the country in the Diamond King's day. In *Step Right Up*, the most comprehensive work on the subject, Brooks McNamara spins the entertaining sagas of outfits like the Kickapoo Indian Medicine Company, the Oregon Indian Medicine Company, and the Hamlin Wizard Oil Company.

Based in New England and run by John "Doc" Healy and Texas Charlie Bigelow, the Kickapoo company produced the Indian oil Sagwa, Kickapoo Buffalo Salve, cough cure, worm killer, and so on. Inventing fantastic stories of frontier adventure for their medicine men's bios, the company kept large troupes of performers on the road throughout the 1880s and 1890s. Often the shows resembled the Wild West extravaganzas staged by Buffalo Bill and other stars of the frontier. McNamara notes that many included "a heavy dose of vaudeville and blackface minstrelsy thrown in for good measure." Other medicine shows featured a pitchman with an Oriental persona, such as the "Hindoo Patalka" show by Dr. N. T. "Nevada Ned" Oliver, which featured Ned "sporting an elaborate buckskin outfit, two Syrians hired out of a rug store, a Hindu who had been doing a vaudeville magic act, and a borrowed elephant which ended the tour by crashing through the floor of a bridge in New Jersey."

Quaker personas were also popular on the med-show circuit—who would fail to trust a pitchman who thou-ed and thee-ed while making a sale? However, Native American imagery seems to have carried the most punch. Although white Americans did indeed obtain genuine medical knowledge from American Indians, as James Harvey Young points out in "Patent Medicines and Indians," American culture exaggerated the Indian's secret medical knowledge for promotional purposes.

Thus, writes Young, "Pocahontas blessed a bitters and Hiawatha helped a hair restorer...Edwin Eastman got a blood syrup from the Comanches, Texas Charlie a panacea from the Kickapoo, and Frank Cushing—a Smithsonian ethnologist, he—a stomach renovator from the Zuni. Besides these notable accretions to pharmacy, there were Modoc Oil, Seminole Cough Balm, Nez Perce Catarrh Snuff, and scores more, all doubtless won for the use of white men by dint of great cunning and valor."

Dr. Frank "White Beaver" Powell observed the marketing power of the Indian mystique while performing with Buffalo Bill and Winnebago Indians in stage plays that predated the big Wild West show. In a related twist on the Cody story, at least one historian believes that Dr. William DeVeny, a pioneer Portland chiropodist and Cody lookalike, may have impersonated the showman at a number of official Buffalo Bill appearances. Cody scholars dismiss the notion, but a reputed photograph of Buffalo Bill with the goateed, buckskinned "Scientific Chiropodist" reveals a startling similarity.

Medicine shows went to great lengths to ensure a theatrical aura that would hold viewers' attention—exotic characters and costumes, spellbinding pitches, mysterious placards, and biological displays. Faith healers of the same era, however, exerted little more than their own presence to charge the landscape about them with a dramatic energy that created great excitement. Don Pedro Jaramillo in Texas, Francis Schlatter in Colorado and New Mexico, Teresa Urrea in Mexico, Arizona, Texas, and California—all felt called by some voice or force to devote their labors to healing the sick with unusual methods that required of the patient steadfast trust.

Whether one believes or disbelieves the stories of their mysterious cures, the three healers, and many others like them, proved that hope and faith can be powerful remedies. Great crowds formed wherever they went. Many who believed they had been helped assisted their natural recovery with a positive attitude. And in some cases, allopathic physicians referred to the healers those patients whose maladies were beyond their means.

To be sure, there were charlatans who offered similar treatments. Robert Karolevitz writes of "strange mystics like Bill the Healer, who operated in Wyoming during the 1870s." Bill would appear in a previ-

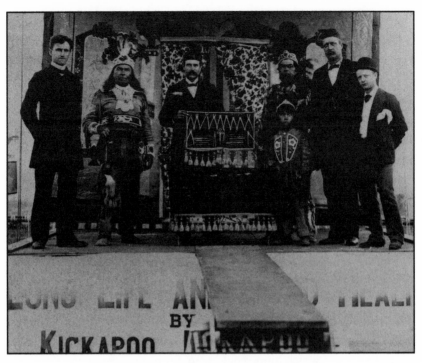

Kickapoo Indian Medicine Company performers.
Photo courtesy Minnesota Historical Society.

ously-unworked saloon, where his planted accomplice would fall deathly ill. Then Bill would step forward, apply his "magic touch," and the shill was miraculously healed. Astounded, the local whiskey drinkers would line up to have Bill lay hands on their lumbago and rheumatism. And Bill would reap big stacks of gold, silver, and greenbacks.

Other, more sincere figures like Jacob "Indian John" Derringer and George Halleck Center combined uncanny perceptual skills with herbal medicine and customized methods of spiritual healing. Akin to parts of their stories was the career of Dr. James W. Gay of Winfield, Kansas. The "Indian Herbal Specialist" advertised in Kansas newspapers early in the twentieth century that he "Tells What Ails You At Sight." The text of an ad from an unnamed newspaper preserved in *Kansas Scrapbook Biography*—accompanied by an engraving of Gay with long hair, wearing fringed buckskin and prairie sombrero, and holding a stalk of some medicinal plant—stated that he "was born in the Miami Village on the Wabash River" in 1840. His Scottish father had practiced medicine among "the Miami and Delaware Nations and the white settlers along the Wabash," where he met Gay's half-Miami mother. At fourteen, the ad continued, Gay "followed the Setting Sun and joined the Pawnees on the Missouri River."

He was wounded three times as he rode into battle with the tribe against the Sioux. And he "commenced the practice of medicine while with the Pawnees, using the knowledge of herbal medicines which [he] had obtained from [his] father." Gay continued his practice back home in Illinois, where he returned to attend school. During the Civil War, he was captured at the Battle of Shiloh and imprisoned at Andersonville. Though losing seventy-three pounds in that "Southern Hell," he states in the ad that he continued practicing medicine. "Even while in prison I prevailed upon the Negroes to bring me certain barks and roots, and with these I cured much sickness and healed many gangrenous wounds. My pay was the gratitude of the poor suffering soldiers."

After the turn of the century, Gay moved from Gladstone, Illinois, to Winfield, Kansas, concluding "to retire from active practice, but to put my celebrated remedies before the public...." After a brief treatise on "universal freedom," which hints that Gay might have encountered resistance to his practice, his ad defends the botanic method with a passage from Ezekiel (47:12): "And by the river upon the bank thereof on this side and on that side shall grow all trees, and the fruit thereof shall be for meat, and the leaf thereof for medicine. For the Lord has created medicines out of the earth and those that are wise will not abhor them."

Newspapers throughout the West carried ads for Chinese and other Asian herbalists in the late nineteenth and early twentieth centuries. As authorities increased licensing restrictions, Asian practitioners encountered greater prejudice. In Phoenix, for instance, former San Francisco herbalist Ah Yeng was arrested in 1897 for practicing medicine without a license. The case's outcome is unknown, but fifteen months later a healer named Ah Yim was serving Phoenix with his Chinese Tea and Herb Sanitarium.

Dr. Ah Fong Chuck emigrated from China, arriving in southeastern Idaho during the gold rush of the 1860s. As Louise Shadduck notes in *Doctors with Buggies, Snowshoes, and Planes*, a California immigration officer inadvertently switched the classically-trained herbalist's name on documents to Chuck Ah Fong. In Idaho, he became known as Dr. C. K. Ah Fong, finding "a ready and willing clientele among both Chinese and

Caucasians in the mining towns." (It was not unusual for culturally-engrained racial prejudice to be overcome in matters of health, as illustrated by the career of Dr. Mud, a part-Indian, part-black healer who ministered to mixed races in Sour Lake, Texas, from the early 1880s to 1903.) After the mines played out in the 1880s, the doctor moved his thriving practice to Boise. When the Idaho State Medical Association was formed in the 1890s, Dr. Fong applied for a license, which was denied. Unintimidated, the Chinese herbalist took the association to court, won his case, and received Idaho's 106th medical license. As Shadduck notes, he was "the only Chinese practitioner to achieve that distinction in the history of Idaho and, at that time, it is believed in the United States."

Sidney A. Weltmer, R. G. Milling, and other "drugless doctors" of the nineteenth and early twentieth centuries even shirked the plant remedies of "nature's pharmacy." Their treatments depended greatly on the healer's personal charisma and his ability to remove obstruction to the flow of a sufferer's "universal life force." Weltmer-inspired individuals set up healing institutes in Emporia, Kansas, Jacksboro, Texas, and other far-flung locations all over the country. The developers of chiropractic and osteopathic medicine practiced the magnetic system before refining their own. In *The Way to Health without Drugs or the Knife,* R. G. Milling described his method as a combination of "Scientific Massage" with the fruits of "sciences or religious sects known as Mesmerism, Hypnotism, Personal Magnetism, Magnetism, Magnetic Healing, Mental Science, Christian Science, Spiritualism, Clairvoyance, Clairaudience, Telepathy, Mediumship, etc."

"The illustrious Oscar Dalton Weeks, celebrated California specialist"—as Frances E. Quebbeman described him in *Medicine in Territorial Arizona*—combined several nineteenth-century medical approaches into an overall system that is difficult to pin down. His diploma from the American Health College of Cincinnati authorized him to "preach and heal with Spiritual Powers and Religious Process, Develope [*sic*] Prophecy and Higher Communion, and to solemnize Marriage, according to law, and to attend funerals."

Weeks traveled the Arizona circuit in the 1890s, "preaching with magnetic power, healing, and selling medicines," through Yavapai, Maricopa, Gila, Cochise, Navajo, and Coconino counties. In Benson and Solomonville, local officials had him arrested despite his diploma and membership in the Vitapathic Society. Arizonans were not shy about expressing their bewilderment with his treatments.

"A burly Irishman struck Doctor Weeks in the face in Clifton," wrote Quebbeman. "During his sojourn in Globe, a dissatisfied patient pulled a gun on the doctor. The patient was arrested," but the doctor and his partner skipped town rather than testify. "No more was heard of Doctor Weeks in Arizona Territory."

Even those physicians whose treatments might have been more aligned with the "regulars"—such as the surgical practice of Dr. Sofie Herzog and the X-ray therapy of Father Kroeger—were required to exhibit creativity and impromptu innovation. Often, the bewildering array of treatment choices and the stresses of a frontier medical practice drove a pioneer doctor to drown his misery in the bottle. Sometimes the medicine man swilled his own "snake oil," heavily fortified with alcohol "for medicinal value only." An example of the type, the silk-hatted, traveling tonic pitchman in Sam Shepard's film *Silent Tongue* seems to have consumed the majority of his inventory.

In an 1880 letter to his brother, quoted in *Step Right Up*, med-show novice Donald McKay wrote: "Last night our long hair Dr had to git drunk and Raze hell and sum Fellow gave him a Belt on the nose and laid the indin Doctor Flat on the Floor with his long hair all over his Fase and this Morning thair Was a long Peas in the Paper. ...Kit has bad luck with his indin Doctors he had a Man name Dr yella Stone and he ran away With Carson dimond pin that cost Five Hundred and Fifty Dollars."

Owen Tully Stratton had the same problem with a Dr. Park, who handled the "office cases" referred to him by pitchman Stratton when the pair toured their low-budget medicine show through Montana, Idaho, Nevada, and West Coast states in the late nineteenth and early twentieth centuries. When stewed, the sixtyish Dr. Park, described by Stratton in his memoir as looking like "a substantial gentleman of the old school," sat in the younger man's hotel room "broke, dirty, smeared with tobacco juice," about to suffer "an attack of the katzenjammers."

Knowing he had to keep Dr. Park at least partly on the wagon for the troupe to succeed, Stratton bought a bottle of whiskey and "doled it out in homeopathic doses." This kept the doctor "almost on an even keel" for a time. Interestingly, Stratton was one of the few med-show performers who left the "snake oil" show business for an accredited medical school, graduating from Barnes Medical College in St. Louis in 1906 and practicing "regular" medicine for several decades.

If Stratton, who grew up in Litchfield, Illinois, attended the World's Columbian Exposition in Chicago in 1893, he might have seen a famed purveyor on the snake-oil scene, Clark Stanley the Rattlesnake King. While some medicine promoters believed the term "snake oil" to be an insult, Stanley made it the name of his nostrum. At the fair, the Texas cowboy-turned-medicine man held crowds breathless and bug-eyed at his rattlesnake-killing booth. Attired in picturesque western garb, he methodically slaughtered hundreds of the notorious reptiles and processed the juices into his quick-selling, sure-cure Snake Oil Liniment.

At least that's how he tells it in his curious pamphlet *The Life and Adventures of the American Cowboy or True Life in the Far West by Clark Stanley, Better Known as the Rattlesnake King.* First published in 1897, various editions of the booklet include the King's life story, some peculiar information on cowboy life, lyrics for cowboy songs, and advertisements for Stanley's White Cactus Soap, Western Herbs, and the old standby Clark Stanley's Snake Oil Liniment, said to be "good for man and beast."

Though the town wasn't founded until long after he was born, Stanley claimed to hail from Abilene, Texas. A cowboy for eleven years, the Rattlesnake King made his first trip up the cattle trail at age fourteen. In the spring of 1879, the tale continues, he traveled to the Arizona settlement of Wolpi [Walpi?] to witness the Snake Dance of the Moki Pueblo.

"There," the Rattlesnake King explained, "I became acquainted with the medicine man of the Moki tribe, and as he liked the looks of my Colt revolver…I gave him an exhibition of my fancy shooting, which pleased him very much." After witnessing the dramatic Snake Dance, the young cowboy was so impressed he stayed with the Indians for thirty months.

He learned their language and dances and the secret of making their medicines. The remedy that interested him most was their Snake Oil Medicine, as he stated the Indians called it, which they used for rheumatism, colds, and all other aches and pains.

"As I was thought a great deal of by the medicine man, he gave me the secret of making the Snake Oil Medicine," Stanley related. He promptly named it Clark Stanley's Snake Oil Liniment. "Snake Oil is not a new discovery," he wrote. "It has been in use by the Mokis and other Indian tribes for many generations, and I have made improvements on the original formula."

Taking leave of the Mokis, Stanley returned to Abilene and unleashed the wonders of Snake Oil Liniment on a rheumatism epidemic. Folks perked up so much that the cowboy began manufacturing in bulk and hit the road to hawk the elixir.

At the Chicago fair, eastern druggists lured him to Providence, Rhode Island, where he established a factory to produce Snake Oil Liniment and his other products. Some snakes were reportedly raised in Rhode Island, but most were shipped to the factory from his snake farm back in Texas.

Most likely, of course, Stanley's ingredients came from eastern manufacturers who'd never been within three states of a Texas rattler. Federal chemists examined a seized shipment of the liniment in 1917 and found it to be a light mineral oil mixed with about 1 percent of fatty oil (probably beef fat), red pepper, and possibly a trace of camphor and turpentine. It is also possible, if not likely, that Stanley never saw the Moki Snake Dance. Still, visions of exotic ceremonies in the faraway land of Arizona must have enchanted metropolitan dwellers as they read of thrilling western adventures in the Rattlesnake King's booklet while soothing their neuralgia and lumbago with Snake Oil Liniment.

Some Indian tribes, such as the Choctaws, did use rattlesnake grease as a liniment for rheumatism. Other cultures valued the folk remedy as well. Frost Woodhull collected several such usages in *Southwestern Sheep and Goat Raiser* in December 1940. Jovita Gonzales of Del Rio told Woodhull about rattlesnake oil applications for colic, toothache, rheumatism, "suppression of bad instincts," small pox marks, and for fits and convulsions. "When applied to the hair (as brilliantine) of frivolous, coquettish young ladies," reported Woodhull, snake oil "will pacify their turbulent instincts. This can be done only when the moon is on the wane, otherwise the result will be quite the opposite."

Willis Woolens, curator of San Antonio's Snake Garden, told Woodhull anecdotes of snake oil cures of a mule's deafness and a milk cow's sore, chapped teats. Another tale contends that a snake oil treatment for a dog's mange resulted in creation of the Mexican hairless breed. Woolens once shined his boots with rattler oil; while riding his horse to town that day, he discovered a pack of one hundred javelinas following, thinking they'd scented a tasty meal of snake meat.

Like many (if not most) of the medical treatments administered by the individuals in this book, snake oil, though regarded as quackery, did often improve a consumer's health. What a surprise it would be for Clark Stanley to discover that rattlesnake venom is today used by biotech researchers in an effort to clone proteins that may someday help retard the growth of tumors in the human body.

BIBLIOGRAPHIC ESSAY

Works consulted include *Doctors of the American Frontier* by Richard Dunlop (Garden City, N.Y.: Doubleday, 1965); *Doctors of the Old West: A Pictorial History of Medicine on the Frontier* by Robert Karolevitz (New York: Bonanza Books, 1967); *Gold Fever* by George Groh (New York: William Morrow, 1966); *Step Right Up* by Brooks McNamara (Jackson: University of Mississippi Press, 1995); *Doctors with Buggies, Snowshoes, and Planes* by Louise Shadduck (Boise, Id.: Tamarack Press, 1993); *Medicine in Territorial Arizona* by Frances E. Quebbeman (Phoenix: Arizona Historical Foundation, 1966); Clark Stanley's *The Life and Adventures of the American Cowboy or True Life in the Far West by Clark Stanley, Better Known as the Rattlesnake King* (Providence, R.I.: Clark Stanley, 1897); *William Money: A Southern California Savant* by William B. Rice (Los Angeles: n.p., 1943); "The Remarkable Qualities of Rattlesnake Oil" by Frost Woodhull, published in *Southwestern Sheep and Goat Raiser* (December 1940); and *The Way to Health without Drugs or the Knife* by R. G. Milling (Cisco, Tex.: Hotel Milling Sanitarium, 1917).

Dr. James W. Gay appears briefly in *Medicine in Kansas, 1850–1900* by Larry Jochims (Emporia, Kans.: Emporia State University Research Studies, 1981), and at greater length in *Kansas Scrapbook Biography* 6, Kansas State Historical Society, Topeka.

Viola Lockhart Warren wrote about "Medical Quacks and Heroes of Early California" in *Southern California Quarterly* (June 1959). Nancy "Grandma" Parker information is on file at the Texas Historical Commission. "The Daughters of Shiprah, Folk Healers and Midwives of the Great Plains" by Timothy J. Kloberdanz appeared in *Great Plains Quarterly* (Winter 1989). "Folk Medicine" by Don Yoder appears in *Folklore and Folklife*, edited by Richard Dotson (Chicago: University of Chicago Press, 1972). Dr. Henry F. Hoyt chronicled his medical adventures in *A Frontier Doctor* (Boston: Houghton Mifflin, 1929). Hoyt ranged from Deadwood, South Dakota, to the Texas Panhandle and Bernalillo and Las Vegas, New Mexico. In the last locales he utilized adobe splints and survived run-ins with Billy the Kid and Jesse James. "Patent Medicines and Indians" by James Harvey Young appeared in *Emory University Quarterly* (Summer 1961). Don Holm told the Dr. DeVeny story in "Were There Two Buffalo Bills?" (*Frontier Times*, August/September 1965). The rollicking memoir of Owen Tully Stratton was published as *Medicine Man* (Norman: University of Oklahoma Press, 1989).

The most reliable, comprehensive text on genuine Indian healing may be *American Indian Medicine* by Virgil J. Vogel (Norman: University of Oklahoma Press, 1970). For a good capsulization and survey of the various systems of American medicine and their development, see *The Great American Medicine Show, Being an Illustrated History of Hucksters, Healers, Health Evangelists and Heroes from Plymouth Rock to the Present* by David Armstrong and Elizabeth Metzger Armstrong (New York: Prentice Hall, 1991). Patent medicine collector A. Walker Bingham provides an enjoyable, well-illustrated survey of the industry's advertising in *The Snake Oil Syndrome* (Hanover, Mass.: The Christopher Publishing House, 1994.)

Francis Schlatter: The Healer of the Southwest

FERENC M. SZASZ

The photographic division of the Library of Congress contains several stereo-cards of a remarkable scene. It was the fall of 1895, and over a thousand people were lined up in Denver to be touched by a German immigrant who bore a startling resemblance to pictures of Jesus. They would walk up to a wooden platform, grasp the hands of the man—who would offer a short prayer—and then walk away. Many testified to miraculous cures. Moreover, the man took no payment. "I have no use for money," he said. Whenever people thanked him, he replied, "Don't thank me; thank the Heavenly Father. Put your faith in him, not in me. I have no power but what he gives me through my faith. He will give you the same." The man was Francis Schlatter (1856–1897), "The New Mexico Messiah," "The Healer," "El Gran Hombre," and his is one of the most remarkable stories of the Southwest during the 1890s.

Francis Schlatter was born on April 29, 1856, in the French province of Alsace-Lorraine. His parents were German peasants, and he quit school at fourteen to learn the trade of a shoemaker. Born a Roman Catholic, he remained one throughout his life. When his parents died, he immigrated to America, where he arrived around 1884. He spent several years in New York City and in Jamesport, Long Island, working both as a shoemaker and as a fireman on the local steamboats. Then, in the fall of 1892 he came to Denver and established a business, first on Stout Street and later on Downing Avenue.

While working at his trade in Denver, Schlatter cured a friend through advice in a letter. As a result of this, he began to feel that "The Father" had chosen him to perform great deeds of healing. First, however, he felt he would have to be tested. Consequently, in July of 1893 he left Denver in the rain, with only $3 in his pocket, and began to wander

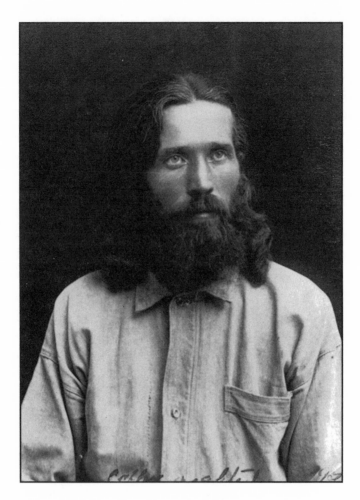

Francis Schlatter, known as The New Mexico Messiah, The Healer, and El Gran
Hombre, drew national attention in the 1890s with remarkable healings in
New Mexico and Colorado.
Photo by Albright Art Studio, courtesy Museum of New Mexico, neg. no. 51264.

across the western United States. He had no itinerary but simply followed the voice of The Father.

His wanderings lasted almost two years. From Denver he walked through Kansas, stopping at Clay Center, Topeka, and Lawrence. At Kansas City, he turned south, where he eventually entered Indian Territory. When he came to Hot Springs, Arkansas, he was arrested for vagrancy, given fifty lashes, and thrown in jail for five months. After he was released, he traveled through Texas, where he was again arrested at Throckmorton and spent three more days in jail. From there he went to El Paso, across the desert to Yuma, and finally to San Diego. He began healing in the San Diego area during July 1894 (where he was robbed by a fellow wanderer). Then he journeyed to San Francisco, eventually crossing the Mojave Desert, and rested a few months while herding sheep with some Navajo Indians around Flagstaff, Arizona. Since he had little money, he either begged food or did without. Although friendly railroad men offered him rides on occasion, he walked most of the way, usually barefoot. His fellow itinerants poked fun at "that crazy shoemaker," as they called him, but they were also in awe of him.

Schlatter arrived in Pajarito, New Mexico, a hamlet near present-day Los Lunas, around July 9, 1895. Drawing on the *curandero* tradition of the little Spanish village, he began healing there in earnest. Stories of numerous cures soon reached Albuquerque, and the *Albuquerque Morning Democrat* sent reporters to investigate. In Los Lunas they encountered incredible tales of healing—stories that would have been instantly dismissed if hundreds of people had not vouched for their truth. For example, Jesus Maria Vasques, who had been blind for three years, was touched by Schlatter and now could see. Juliana Sedillo, who had not been able to use her arms for sixteen years, was now off working in the fields, and so on. One person who confirmed the stories was Andreas Romero, an elderly, prominent citizen of nearby Peralta. "The work of this man is something inexplicable and wonderful," he told the *Albuquerque Morning Democrat* on July 17. "There is something in his touch which seels to heal the sick. What you have heard of him is true to the letter. I cannot explain it myself; no one can; yet we know some remarkable cures have been effected." When the paper broke the story, the issue sold out immediately. "El Sanador" became the principal topic of conversation on every street corner.

In addition to his healing, the mystery surrounding Schlatter deepened when he confessed to reporters that The Father had instructed him to fast and that he had eaten nothing for over ten days. The people with whom he was living vouched for this. "Food is not necessary to him who has the proper faith in my Master," he told the *Albuquerque Morning Democrat.* The people of Albuquerque were surprised when he ended his fast by eating a gigantic meal and seemingly felt no ill after-effects. Stranger still, Schlatter bore an uncanny resemblance to the standard representations of Jesus. The *Albuquerque Morning Democrat* reporter gulped as his gaze moved from Schlatter to an inexpensive print of Christ on the wall behind him. "As one looked from the flesh to the presentment [on the wall]," he noted, "the likeness was startling. Every line and touch to be found in the picture were found in the man." Moreover, observers were astounded when, after being specifically asked, Schlatter informed Reverend Charles Bovard that he was Jesus returned for a second life on earth.

Following the newspaper reports on Schlatter, the people of Albuquerque urged him to cole to their city, and he arrived there on July 20. His fame had preceded him, and when he began healing in Old Town the following day he was met by a huge crowd. Here, however, he encountered his first opposition. "The Catholic Church does not sanction or approve of such proceedings," said Albuquerque priest Father Mandalari in the July 21 *Albuquerque Morning Democrat.* "He is a fraud from beginning to end," remarked trader Frank A. Hubbell a day later to the paper's reporters. A prominent judge said he should probably be locked up under the vagrancy act. Yet none of the local police would have dared to arrest him, so convinced were the people of his power. "The train of wagons which never seems to end," noted the July 23 *Albuquerque Morning Democrat,* "prove better than argument the implicit faith the people have in the strange man."

Numerous people claimed to have been healed, and in spite of careful scrutiny no one was able to detect fraud in any of the reported cures: Black railroad worker Charles Stamp could suddenly walk on his crushed foot; Peter Maguire found himself cured of his rheumatism; Mrs. C. J. Roentgen could now hear better; and C. G. Lott could suddenly move his paralyzed arm. To those who felt no improvement, Schlatter simply said that more treatments were necessary. Moreover, he continued to refuse payment for his work; when money was occasionally forced on him, he later distributed it to the poor. Schlatter was always very open whenever he was questioned about his power. He was only a poor shoemaker, he said, who was simply doing the bidding of his Master. When the July 27 *Albuquerque Weekly Citizen* asked him to account for the cures, he replied, "My work speaks for itself."

By the middle of August, Schlatter's fame had spread across the Rocky Mountain West. Edward L. Fox, a former Denver alderman who had come to Albuquerque with an ill friend, was able to convince Schlatter to go to Denver; according to the August 12 *Santa Fe Daily New Mexican* and the August 11 *Albuquerque Morning Democrat*, he made plans to leave on August 21. "How long will you be in Denver?" a reporter asked him. "Not over two months," was the reply. "Where will you go then?" "No one knows but The Father," said Schlatter. "Probably I will disappear and no one will know where I am." "Will you return ever?" "Yes," he said, "but not in the form that I have now."

Weak and somewhat ill from his efforts, Schlatter rested in several prominent Albuquerque homes until time to depart for Denver. Numerous citizens, including the merchants, were very sorry to see him go, for he had brought many people into the city. A crowd gathered at the station to see him off, and many wept openly when he boarded the train. When the train stopped at Bernalillo, Cerrillos, Lamy, Las Vegas, and on up the line on its way north, people crowded the platforms for a glimpse of Schlatter or a word from him. Whenever Schlatter emerged from the coach, he told the crowds that it was not necessary that he touch them to effect healing. The Father would cure them of their ills, he said, because their coming to the station was proof of their faith. "Last night," noted an *Albuquerque Morning Democrat* reporter, "the curtain dropped on a drama which will claim a place in the history of the Territory of New Mexico."

In Denver Schlatter rested for several weeks at the E. L. Fox home. During that time, Fox had a special platform built behind his house so that the crowds could come up single file and be touched. On September 16, Schlatter again began healing. Typically, he would start at 9:00 A.M. and work until 5:00 P.M. At times he would walk among the crowds and touch invalids who could not mount the platform. Often he blessed handkerchiefs that were held up to him. One reporter guessed that six people passed him every minute; some crowds were estimated at three thousand. Schlatter ministered in this manner, with no rest, for almost two months.

The people of Denver were as amazed as the people of Albuquerque had been. Streetcars were crowded with the faithful, the scoffers, and the merely curious. Lines began to form before dawn, and during the day small boys moved among them selling iced drinks, popcorn, and sandwiches. Some entrepreneurs arrived early in order to sell their places in line to latecomers. Those who claimed they had been cured spread the word to friends and acquaintances. For example, when an official of the Union Pacific Railroad was cured of deafness, he offered his employees free trips to Denver. Special trains also ran from Albuquerque and Omaha. Moreover, so many people tried to withdraw their children from the Colorado Springs State Institute for the Deaf and Blind that the officials sought (unsuccessfully) to have Schlatter visit their institution. The story was even carried in eastern papers. "The work of this man of faith," remarked one reporter for the *Santa Fe Daily New Mexican,* "is one of the greatest sensations in Denver for years."

Denunciations by Denver's doctors and clergymen proved no match for the testimonials of miraculous cures. Despite persistent scoffing by some people, many cures were verified by outsiders. Several people signed affidavits, while other cures were attested to by skeptical reporters. "Faith moveth mountains," remarked Joseph Emerson Smith, who covered the story for the *Denver Post.* Forty-six years later, Smith told the *Empire Magazine,* "I am still unable to account otherwise for the healings I saw."

Some unscrupulous individuals attempted to make money from this excitement by selling handkerchiefs (supposedly blessed by Schlatter) as far away as the East Coast. However, the federal government indicted them for using the mails to defraud and had plans to call Schlatter as a witness against them. But before any action could be taken Schlatter disappeared. On the morning of November 14, 1895, as Thomas F. Dawson wrote in *The Trail,* Fox and his wife went to wake the healer, only to find a note pinned to the pillow of his cot: "Mr. Fox—My mission is finished. Father takes me away. Goodbye, [signed] Francis Schlatter."

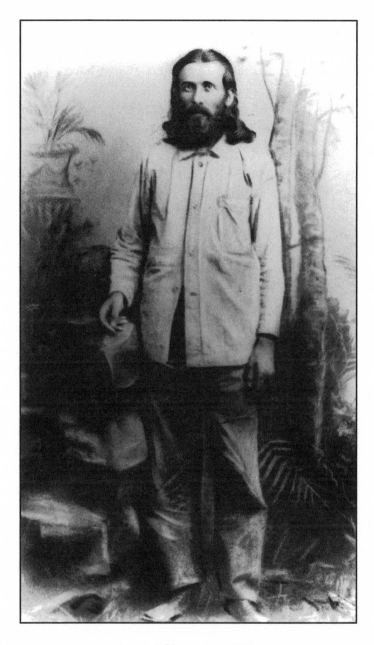

Francis Schlatter, circa 1895.
Photo by Albright Art Studio, courtesy Museum of New Mexico,
neg. no. 132505.

Subsequently, the Denver papers began a hunt for Schlatter as if he were public enemy number one. Sightings were reported in every area of the state as well as in Kansas City and Omaha. The hundreds of people who had come to see him voiced their disappointment, and souvenir hunters tore down the fence surrounding Fox's house. Meanwhile, Schlatter was slowly riding south into New Mexico on his big white horse, Butte.

In mid-December Schlatter was spotted in the Santa Fe area, and he spent time healing in Pena Blanca, Santo Domingo, and Bernalillo. Although several prominent citizens urged him to return to Albuquerque, he refused to commit himself. He would go where The Father wished, he said. When word of his whereabouts spread, numerous packages and letters were sent to him care of the postmaster of Santa Fe. "Suffering humanity outside of New Mexico," remarked an editor of the *Santa Fe Daily New Mexican,* "is trying hard to definitely locate Schlatter, the healer."

Early in January Schlatter quietly appeared at the Morley Ranch in Datil (near Socorro). There he met a sympathetic listener, Mrs. Ada Morley (Jarrett), who gladly housed him for the winter months. "The Father has directed me to a safe retreat," he told her, according to Agnes Morley Cleaveland. "I must restore my spiritual powers in seclusion and prayer." For three months Schlatter remained secluded in an upstairs room at the Morley household, venturing out only when there was no one around. During that time he alternately rested and exercised by swinging a large copper rod over his head, as a drum major might swing a baton. He said that The Father had told him this was necessary or he would lose his power. He and Mrs. Morley had long conversations during the winter, and, with his permission, she copied them down. In this manuscript Schlatter elaborated on his views of The Father, his impressions of the truth of reincarnation, his criticism of American society, and his vision of the coming New Jerusalem. Later the book was published as *The Life of the Harp in the Hand of the Harper,* only three copies of which are still extant. Historians owe a great debt of gratitude to Mrs. Morley since this little book provides the only reliable source for Schlatter's ideas and social attitudes.

When spring arrived, Schlatter informed his hostess that it was time for him to leave. Word had leaked out as to his whereabouts, and people were beginning to seek his aid at the ranch. After bidding Mrs. Morley goodbye, he headed south. He was spotted near Silver City on April 8, but he apparently avoided most settled areas. He crossed the border into Mexico a few days later.

For over twenty years afterward, imposters claiming to be Schlatter appeared intermittently across the nation. Chicago, New York City, Canton, Ohio, central Nebraska, Los Angeles, Long Beach, and St. Louis all produced healers who said they were he. But there was a key difference between Schlatter and his imposters: they almost always took money.

Schlatter himself lived only about a year after he left the Morley Ranch. He died sometime in 1897 in Chihuahua, Mexico. Rumors of his death spread in the spring of 1897, but they were discounted by his followers. His passing was reported in 1901 by H. F. Gray, a Los Angeles doctor, a report confirmed five years later by archaeologist Edgar L. Hewett. Hewett tells it this way: In the spring of 1906, he was surveying the eastern slope of the Sierra Madres, near Casas Grandes, about 150 miles south of the American border. Here he heard the story of Schlatter's death from his Mexican guide. Several years earlier the guide had found a white horse standing by a man he assumed was sleeping. When he ran to get the village authorities, they discovered that the man was dead. "Francis Schlatter" was written on the flyleaf of the Bible in the saddlebags, and a large copper rod lay nearby. After Hewett donated a check to the village educational fund, the *jefe politico* of Casas Grandes gave him the rod. Hewett, in turn, donated it to the Museum of New Mexico, where it is today. Thus, while much of the western United States was seeking Schlatter, the healer had quietly passed away in a tiny Mexican village.

Francis Schlatter was not the first American to heal by faith, of course, and numerous twentieth-century healers have continued this tradition. Kathryn Kuhlman of Minneapolis, Oral Roberts of Tulsa, the "psychic surgeons" of the Philippine Islands, and numerous lesser-known Pentecostals are still very much in evidence. However, Schlatter's career reflects the time in which he lived—a period which could be considered an "age of transition" in American culture. Major changes were occurring in two areas especially: the relationship between rich and poor and the world of medicine.

Historians agree that the "Gay Nineties" hardly deserve their sobriquet since the depression which lasted from 1893 to 1897—without any governmental intervention—may well have been the nation's worst. The violent strikes at Homestead, Pennsylvania (1892), and Pullman, Illinois (1894), were only the most spectacular of thousands of smaller labor-management conflicts. The election of 1896, which pitted Democrat and Populist William Jennings Bryan against Republican William McKinley, saw America deeply divided along economic lines. In 1892, Episcopal priest John J. McCook estimated that there were perhaps 50,000 unemployed men roaming the land. One of them—Connecticut Fatty—told McCook that there were only two truly happy people in the world—the millionaire and the bum. During the 1890s there were plenty of both.

Schlatter can best be understood as a product of the social unrest of the 1890s. He denounced American society for its love of money and for its injustice to the working classes. "The moneyed few," he stated in *The Life of the Harp in the Hand of the Harper*, "are the bloodsucking parasites on the common people." Moreover, he interpreted the message of Jesus as utopian socialism. He told Mrs. Morley:

> Never forget I was a workingman. It's a devilish system! It's the cursed institution and those who uphold it will reap their reward. If they sow the wind they will reap the whirlwind. That is the law from on high. Have they clothed the naked, fed the hungry? Have they housed the homeless? Have they protected the widow and orphan?
>
> There has been no peace since Adam. Is not 6,000 years enough? How long must they suffer? But the day cometh when the promises for thousands of years shall be fulfilled. He will show the world unmistakably that He is the Lord their God and they are His people. Then we shall have peace, once and forever.

Yet Schlatter was not a political person; he despaired of political solutions. According to him, it would serve no purpose to give women the franchise; it would do no good to vote for the Populists. It was too late. The end of time was approaching. Schlatter predicted that in 1899 there would be a terrible war between the wealthy and the laboring classes. (He missed the McKinley-Bryan election by only three years.)

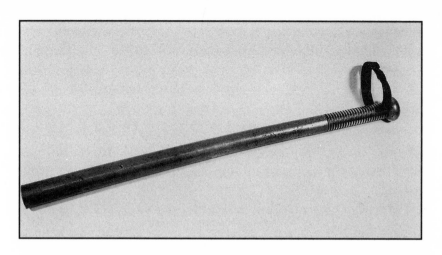

Francis Schlatter's copper "healing rod."
Courtesy Museum of New Mexico, neg. no. 67152.

After the confrontation, the Lord would establish a New Jerusalem in America—located in Datil, New Mexico. Not without reason was Schlatter called "the democrat's Jesus" in *The Life of the Harp in the Hand of the Harper.*

The 1890s were also a great time of transition for American medicine. The age of scientific medicine was dawning, but it had not yet arrived. In *Principles and Practices of Medicine*, the chief textbook of the College of Physicians and Surgeons in New York, Dr. William Osler noted that "modern medicine could cure only four or five diseases." Thanks to the discoveries of Louis Pasteur, Robert Koch, and Joseph Lister, medicine was able to *prevent* many infections—antiseptic measures during surgery could halt infection; clean drinking water could stop the spread of cholera and typhoid; doctors could vaccinate against smallpox; quinine could alleviate malarial fevers. But very few diseases could actually be *cured*—primarily the "deficiency diseases" such as scurvy and beriberi, which could be corrected by proper diet. The miracle drugs of sulfa, penicillin, and the like were all products of the twentieth century.

Although the germ theory of disease had been accepted in most medical circles by the 1880s, medical practitioners did not always adhere to its principles. As late as 1885, Dr. William E. Mayo of Rochester, Minnesota (father of the two famous Mayo brothers), performed surgery without using Lister's antiseptic precautions. And in 1892 a famous German doctor drank a beaker full of cholera bacilli to prove that the germ theory was nonsense. He survived, presumably because he was so angry that his stomach acids killed the bacilli before they could kill him. New ideas in the world of medicine spread slowly.

Moreover, in the 1890s neither New Mexico nor Colorado was at the forefront of medical science. For cures, most people relied on home remedies or the numerous patent medicines that were readily available. The heyday of patent medicines was from 1880 to 1900. Before federal regulation in 1906, these concoctions could, and did, promise anything. While the *Albuquerque Weekly Citizen*, the [Socorro] *Citizen*, and other newspapers wrote skeptically of Schlatter's cures, they simultaneously ran advertisements for Dr. Louden's Cholera Compound ("the only known preventative"); Dr. Miles's Heart Nervine ("permanently cures every kind of nervous disease"); and Dr. McLean's Liver and Kidney Balm (which reminded readers, "You can't live without a liver").

In addition, in the rush to establish medicine on a scientific basis, late nineteenth-century physicians began to ignore the relationship between mind and body. By slighting a connection that medical practitioners had been aware of since antiquity, they created a tremendous gap in the healing process, which was filled by a body of new ideas collectively known as "New Thought." In the East, New Thought was institutionalized as Christian Science; in the Midwest, as John A. Dowie's Zion City, Illinois; in the Far West as Unity and The Church of Divine Science. New Thought ideas were much in evidence during the 1890s.

The origins of New Thought were varied. It borrowed from Swedish mystic Emanuel Swedenborg, from Ralph Waldo Emerson and American Transcendentalism, and, especially, from the Quaker idea of "Christ consciousness" within. New Thought groups differed considerably but all stressed the possibility of altering one's circumstances simply by changing one's ideas toward them, as well as the legitimacy of divine healing. They argued that God is omnipotent and perfect, that man is part of God, and therefore, that there could be no illness if one were in the right relationship with God. As Denver Divine Science Minister Nona Brooks said, as quoted in the *Denver Post* in 1972, "God is everywhere, therefore God is here. God is health. Health is everywhere. Therefore, health is here."

Schlatter drew heavily on New Thought ideas. Although his critics liked to portray him as an ignorant shoemaker, it is clear from his comments that he had read widely in the literature of his time, including New Thought writings (a large box of books he left with his Denver landlord unfortunately disappeared). He was also known to have attended several gatherings of spiritualists when he lived in Denver. Healer Malinda E. Cramer, a founder of the Church of Divine Science, moved to Denver in 1887, and it is likely he knew of her or the Brooks sisters—well-known New Thought figures. Their messages were similar to his. "My mission is to cure the afflicted when The Father directs me," Schlatter told the *Colorado Sun*, "but unless they have faith my efforts are useless. The greater the faith, the quicker they get well. Some have more disease than others. It doesn't come in a day, and it will not go in a day. When The Father doesn't want it they cannot get it. When He sends it, they have it. It all depends upon what He sends. God is the giver of all things."

Did Schlatter really cure people? It is evident that he definitely did cure some individuals who came to see him. Hundreds of claims of cures emerged, many of them signed and verified; not all of these people could have been mistaken. Modern physicians know that confidence in one's doctor is an important part of the healing process. And few people today doubt that suggestion and autosuggestion can indeed eliminate certain symptoms. In addition, several types of hysterias, neuroses, and even certain types of paralyses are directly related to mental attitude.

Were the cures permanent? There is no way of knowing since no follow-up studies were ever done. Since the *source* of the illness sometimes remained unaffected, the symptoms might have moved around the body. For example, a woman cured of headaches might have developed stomach pains a few weeks later. A man who lost the pain in his arm might have developed another in the leg, and so forth. However, real miracles came from the workings of the minds and bodies themselves. Schlatter was well aware that time heals the majority of illnesses. To the many people who felt no instantaneous improvement, he said that the cures were gradual. They came "as faith comes."

Did Schlatter actually reverse such maladies as cancer, permanent blindness, deafness, or tuberculosis? Almost certainly not. Such cures were beyond the medical knowledge of his time, indeed frequently beyond our present-day knowledge. However, Schlatter was not an imposter. As Walter C. Hadley of Albuquerque said to the *Albuquerque Morning Democrat*, he was just as he represented himself—a poor shoemaker doing the bidding of The Father. Although Hadley could not say where Schlatter's power came from, he remarked, "I do know the man is honest in his intentions, consistent in all things, and that he is doing many men good and no man harm."

BIBLIOGRAPHIC ESSAY

This article first appeared in *New Mexico Historical Review* 54, no. 2 (1979). Works consulted include *The Life of the Harp in the Hand of the Harper* by Francis Schlatter (Denver, Colo.: Smith-Brooks, 1897) and *Biography of Francis Schlatter, The Healer, with his Life, Works and Wanderings* by Harry Byron Magill (Denver, Colo.: Schlatter Publishing Co., 1896). "Francis Schlatter: A Fool for God" by Alice Bullock (*El Palacio* 81, 1975) offers a good short synopsis of his career. See also the compilation of Schlatter materials in Norman Cleaveland, ed., *The Healer: The Story of Francis Schlatter* (Santa Fe, N.M.: Sunstone Press, 1989). I would also like to thank the staff of the Western History Department, Denver Public Library, Charles A. Truxillo, and Margaret Connell Szasz for their assistance in the preparation of this article.

An anonymous publication on Schlatter, *The Divine Healer*, appeared in Denver in 1895. That same year, Fitz Mac published "The 'Christ Man' of Denver" in *The Great Divide*. William Keleher wrote of taking his crippled younger brother, Lawrence, to see Schlatter, but with no effect, in his *Memoirs: 1892–1969* (Santa Fe, N.M.: Rydal Press, 1969). William Jones Wallrich wrote a critical account of Schlatter in "'Christ Man' Schlatter," *New Mexico Folklore Record* 4 (1949–1950). Millard T. Everett wrote "Strange Cures Verified by Skeptical Newsmen," *Catholic Register*, August 21, 1941. *Empire Magazine* ran Wesley B. French's "Denver's Mystery Messiah" on September 30, 1951. Gene Fowler (1890–1960) wrote about Schlatter in *Timberline: A Story of Bonfils and*

Tammen (New York: Covici, Friede, 1933), and Thomas Dawson authored "Francis Schlatter—Denver Healer of the '90s" for *The Trail* 11 (October 1918).

Agnes Morley Cleaveland includes a chapter on the healer in *No Life for a Lady* (Boston: Houghton Mifflin, 1941), and Frank McClelland reported on Schlatter's imitators in *Rocky Mountain News,* March 18, 1928. Edgar L. Hewett recounts his experience in Mexico in *Campfire and Trail* (Albuquerque: University of New Mexico Press, 1943).

Other works consulted include *Principles and Practices of Medicine* by William Osler (New York: D. Appleton and Co., 1892); *All Things Are Possible: The Healing and Charismatic Revivals of Modern America* by David Edwin Harrell, Jr. (Bloomington: Indiana University Press, 1975); *Healing: A Doctor in Search of a Miracle* by William A. Nolen, M.D. (Greenwich, Conn.: Fawcett Press, 1974); "The Depression of the Nineties" by Charles Hoffman, *The Journal of Economic History* 16 (1956); *The Social Reform Papers of John James McCook* edited by Adelia Haberski French (Hartford, Conn.: Antiquarian & Landmarks Society, Inc., of Connecticut, 1977); *William Henry Welch and the Heroic Age of American Medicine* by Simon Flexner and James Thomas Flexner (New York: Viking, 1941); *Microbe Hunters* by Paul De Kruff (New York: Harcourt, Brace & World, 1926); *The Story of Medicine* by Kenneth Walker (New York, 1955); *Half a Century of Medical and Public Health Progress* by Aristides A. Moll (Washington, D.C.: Pan American Union, 1940); *A Hundred Years of Medicine* by C. D. Haagensen and Wyndham E. B. Lloyd (New York: Sheridan House, 1943); "Will Medical History Join the American Mainstream?" by John C. Burnham, *Reviews in American History* 6 (1978); *A Short History of Medicine* by Erwin H. Ackerknecht (New York: Roland Press, 1955); *Plagues and Peoples* by William H. McNeil (New York: Anchor Press, 1976); "American Attitudes Toward the Germ Theory of Disease (1860–1880)," *Journal of the History of Medicine* 9 (1954); *Medicine Without Doctors: Home Health Care in American History* by Guenter B. Risse, Ronald L. Numbers, and Judith Walker Leavitt (New York: Science History Publications, 1977); *The Great Patent Medicine Era* by Adelaide Hechtlinger (New York: Grosset & Dunlap, 1970); *The Toadstool Millionaires: A Social History of Patent Medicines in America Before Federal Regulation* by James Harvey Young (Princeton, N.J.: Princeton University Press, 1961); *American Physicians in the Nineteenth Century: From Sects to Science* by William G. Rothstein (Baltimore, Md.: Johns Hopkins University Press, 1972); *Civilization and Disease* by Henry E. Sigerist (Ithaca, N.Y.: Cornell University Press, 1943); *The Medical Profession and Social Reform* by Lloyd C. Taylor, Jr. (New York: St. Martin's, 1974); *A History of Medicine* by Brian Inglis (Cleveland, Ohio: World Publishing Co., 1965); "Divine Science Origins Traced" by Virginia Culver, *Denver Post,* August 19, 1972; *The Body Is the Hero* by Ronald J. Glasser (New York: Random House, 1976).

Teresa Urrea: "The Saint of Cabora"

FRANK BISHOP PUTNAM

On December 15, 1902, the *Los Angeles Times* printed the following item:

FLOCKING TO SEE SANTA TERESA. STREAM OF MEXI-
CANS FLOWING TO HER COTTAGE. YESTERDAY WAS A
BUSY DAY FOR THE YAQUI GIRL, AND TEAMS THAT
CAME FROM AFAR WERE FASTENED AT HER DOOR.

Santa Teresa, the famed Mexican girl from the land of the Yaqui, in
Sonora, who is implicitly believed in by the majority of Mexicans of the
Southwest as a healer, who exercises supernatural powers, has settled in
Los Angeles permanently, her followers say, and is besieged by a pitiful
throng of Mexican Infermos.

The halt, the blind, the inwardly distressed, paralytics almost help-
less, and others ravaged by consumption, are helped to her doors each
day by friends, and relatives, and none go there without the belief that by
the laying on of her magic hands they will be cured.

Teresa has purchased a little cottage at Brooklyn and State Street, and
a stream of invalids visited the healer in her home yesterday. No distance
seems too great for the Mexicans who believe in the magnetic young
woman from the South, and behind her house are drawn up wagons that
have borne cripples from points in Sonora and other districts along the
Mexican line.

Santa Teresa has great power over the Yaquis, from whose country she
sprang, and has been the subject of many fantastic stories based more or
less on fact. In some ways her influence is really remarkable.

If I had not been investigating some labor troubles that occurred in
1902 among the section-hand workers of the Southern Pacific Railroad,

I would not have given the article a second thought. I had learned that one of our chief agitators causing the labor troubles was a young Mexican woman, whose name and background were unknown. Proceeding on the assumption that the labor agitator and "Santa Teresa" were the same person, I started a two-year investigation to determine her background and why she would be a labor agitator. My quest took me to Nogales, Tucson, Phoenix, Safford and Clifton, Arizona, and to Santa Barbara, California, and El Paso, Texas. Although I eventually discovered that there was no connection between the labor agitator and Teresa Urrea, commonly called the "Saint of Cabora," I found Urrea such a fascinating person that I could not stop researching her short but eventful life. The following is a summary of her extraordinary career.

Teresa Urrea (1873–1905) was born in a *ramada,* a little brush arbor, on a ranch near Ocoroni, Sinaloa, Mexico, October 15, 1873. In regard to her family, she said in an interview with the *San Francisco Examiner,* July 27, 1900, "My mother was a very poor Mexican girl. Her name was Cayetana Chavez. My father was well-to-do. His name is Tomas Urrea. I am not a legitimate child. My mother was only fourteen when I was born. My father has eighteen children and my mother has four. Not one of them is my own full brother or sister."

Urrea, known as Teresita to family and friends, along with her child mother Cayetana, lived in the *ramada* of Cayetana's sister, a dominating, tyrannical woman. As Teresita began to crawl on the dirt floor and then walk, her personality and physical traits developed. She was a fair-skinned and beautiful child, contrasting vividly with the dark-skinned children of her aunt, who developed an avid hatred of the illegitimate child of the *patron* of the ranch. When not being tongue-lashed by her aunt, young Urrea was a happy child who played with children of the other workers on the ranch.

Her father, Don Tomas Urrea, was a man of liberal convictions and active in the political affairs of Mexico. In 1876, he backed Sebastian Lerdo de Tejada, a liberal running for reelection as president of Mexico against the conservative, autocratic provincial general Parfirio Díaz. However, an election was never held since Díaz executed a military coup and seized power. Lerdo fled into exile while Díaz began eliminating Lerdo's supporters. Don Tomas realized he must either declare for Díaz or leave the state of Sinaloa.

Don Tomas had married his first cousin, Doña Loreto Esceberri. They had a common uncle, Miguel Urrea, who had silver mines at Alamos, Sonora, and Cinipas, Chihuahua, as well as several cattle ranches in Sonora. As a wedding present Miguel had given them one of the ranches, called Cabora. Rather than support the regime of Díaz, Don Tomas decided to move to this ranch. Miguel, who encouraged him to make the change, offered the couple a large house in Alamos and to sell them two other ranches adjoining Cabora on easy terms. The three ranches were situated about halfway between Alamos and present-day Obregon.

In 1880, Don Tomas moved his family and retainers to the new location. The result was an exodus of a hundred or more people—Teresita and her mother and aunt, families of the vaqueros, field workers, and domestic servants, followed by herds and flocks of animals.

Don Tomas installed Doña Loreto, her children, and her retinue in a large house, called La Capilla, at the edge of Alamos. With his retainers and herds, he moved to the ranch of Santa Maria, which was the one nearest to Alamos—a place he used as a base while he made large-scale improvements at Cabora. The big house at Cabora consisted of wings with broad verandas in front of them, on the north and west sides of a quadrangle 230 feet square. In addition to *ramadas* for workers' families, on the east and south sides were high walls. With a watchtower on the northwest corner the house functioned as a fort as well as an elegant and spacious hacienda headquarters. When the renovations at Cabora were finished and several hundred acres of irrigated farmland had been cultivated, Don Tomas installed a beautiful teenage girl as mistress of Cabora—Gabriela Cantua, who later became his common-law wife. Doña Loreto and her establishment continued to live at La Capilla. During these years, from 1880 to 1888, it is not known at which of the ranches young Urrea and her mother were living.

In an interview with a reporter, which was published in the *San Francisco Examiner,* July 27, 1900, Teresita said, "When I was sixteen my father sent for me to come into his home. I went to his hacienda at Cabora."

From the time she went to Cabora, her story is well known. She was a tall, fragile, graceful girl of great beauty. Fair of skin, with dark chestnut hair, her eyes large and luminous and set far apart, her voice soft and gentle, her presence was compelling. Don Tomas and the entire household at Cabora succumbed to her unaffected charm. She sang and played the guitar, and added spontaneity and zest to the flow of life on the ranch.

Aside from her father, whom she came to adore, the other person on the ranch for whom she developed an attachment and admiration was an old woman, María Sonora, a *curandera*. Teresita became a sort of understudy of Sonora as the old one went on her daily rounds looking after the sick and crippled on the ranch. From Sonora she learned the names of more than a hundred herbs and what maladies they were supposed to cure. Sonora was pleased with the girl's aptitude and began thinking of her as a *curandera* who would succeed her at Cabora. Although it was observed that the girl's presence exerted a strange, hypnotic influence on the sick, something which seemed as beneficial as the herbs, no special attention was given to this phenomenon at the time.

After a few months at Cabora, Teresita suddenly went into a cataleptic state. For fourteen days she was in a deep coma, her body rigid and her heartbeat becoming ever fainter until it seemed to stop entirely. Presumed dead, she was laid out and dressed for burial; a coffin was constructed by the ranch carpenter. An all-night wake was held by the hundreds of people at the ranch. However, late in the night, as women knelt around her saying their prayers, fingering their worn rosaries, Teresita suddenly arose and asked what was going on. A tremendous commotion ensued, and when her father arrived, she told him of a voice that had spoken while she was asleep, telling her she was to help the people. Assuming this was an hallucination due to delirium, her father gave it no further thought, although he was puzzled when she said to him, "The coffin you made for me, we will not need it now, but keep it. María will die in three days. Save it for her." Since he was certain his daughter had no way of knowing about the coffin, this alarmed him, and when María quietly died in her sleep after three days and was buried in the coffin, Don Tomas was troubled.

Following this incident, Teresita was in a trance state for three months. As she later remarked to a reporter from the *San Francisco Examiner*, "For three months and eighteen days, I was in a trance. I know nothing of what I did during that time. They told me, those who saw, that I could move about, but they had to feed me; that I talked strange things about God and religion; that people came to me from all the country around, and if they were sick or crippled, I put my hands on them and they got well. Of this, I remember nothing, but when I came to myself I saw they were well."

A number of legends persist about the first spectacular cure effected by Teresita while she was in a trance. Señora Josefa Soto de Armenta told Dr. and Mrs. Curry Holden and Peter Hurd in April 1957 the first cure was that of a crippled vaquero who had been kicked in the head by a horse several years before. Since that time his limbs and face had been paralyzed on one side. Obsessed with the thought that Teresita could cure him, he appeared before her one day and pleaded with her to heal him. At first she did not know what to do. Then, in desperation she picked up some dirt, mixed it with saliva, and rubbed it on his paralyzed side. According to Soto de Armenta, the cure was instantaneous and complete. Those who witnessed it, shouted, "Miracle, miracle."

News spread through the land that a miracle had occurred at Cabora. By the time Teresita came out of her trance, the roads were filled with people traveling there, and as her power to cure continued, each day the crowds grew larger. Before a year had passed, daily visitors at the ranch numbered in the thousands. A reporter from a newspaper in Las Cruces, New Mexico, gave the number the day he was there at five thousand. During 1890 and 1891, the crowds of pilgrims flocking to the ranch of Cabora became larger and larger. On Teresita's birthday, October 15, 1891, the number was estimated at eight thousand and at Christmas the same year, at ten thousand.

The influx of humanity soon overtaxed the facilities of the ranch. The nearest place supplies could be purchased by the pilgrims was about twenty-five miles away. Although most of them brought food, hundreds had none and had to be fed. Also many rode or drove animals—and these, which later exceeded the number owned by the ranch, needed grass and water.

From the beginning, Don Tomas looked with foreboding on the mounting onrush. At first he had no faith in Teresita's "miracles." He contended the early cures could have been effected by anyone under sufficiently high emotional stress. And he repeatedly urged Teresita to desist and refuse to see the patients. However, in her trance state she was not amenable to logic; and when she was not in a trance state she could not denounce her compassion for the afflicted.

Eventually, Don Tomas resigned himself to the inevitable. He dug more wells to obtain water for the visitors and moved his own cattle to his other ranches. He sold food to pilgrims with money and gave it to those without. In order to keep the crowds away from the big house, he made a room near the blacksmith shop into a chapel and converted a smaller house occupied by an official into a separate residence for Teresita, with an elegance comparable to the big house. Teresita's House, as it quickly became known, had a broad veranda where she received her patients.

A wide range of people from all social and economic strata came to Cabora but mostly the poor. Predominant were the "Christianized" Indians—the Yaquis and Mayos from Sonora, the Gusaves from Sinaloa, and the Tarahumaras from Chihuahua. Nine out of ten pilgrims were barefoot or wore *huaraches*. About the same percentage could not read or write. They believed in the saints and came to witness miracles. They called Teresita *La Niña de Cabora, Santa Teresa,* and *La Santa de Cabora.* She objected vehemently to all these appellations except the first and continuously contended that she was not a saint but an ordinary person with a special gift to be used for the good of humanity—much like a writer or a singer.

On rare occasions, Teresita foretold events that would take place in the future. One day, after recovering from a short trance, a common occurrence, she prophesied that a tornado would strike on an adjoining ranch at a given time. No one took her seriously until the tornado struck precisely when she had said it would. Don Tomas could not understand this faculty of predicting the future—something apparently unconnected to mental mechanisms of association. By contrast, the ability to recall events in the past or attain knowledge of what was happening at a distance could be accounted for by psychological laws of association and mental telepathy.

Moreover, unusual circumstances that had no direct connection with Teresita's curing powers occurred. For instance, the chemistry of her body was such that her perspiration had an odor similar to perfume. When she was tense while effecting a difficult cure, she perspired, and the air around her for some distance was as if sprayed with a delectable fragrance. One day she was aghast when she discovered her maid carefully saving her bathwater and distributing it to a waiting line of women, who took it away to be used for all kinds of healing purposes—believing it contained the "goodness" which exuded from her body.

Teresita's relationship with the Catholic Church became increasingly strained as she was more and more venerated. The hierarchy of the Catholic Church took a dim view of the events at Cabora. Although

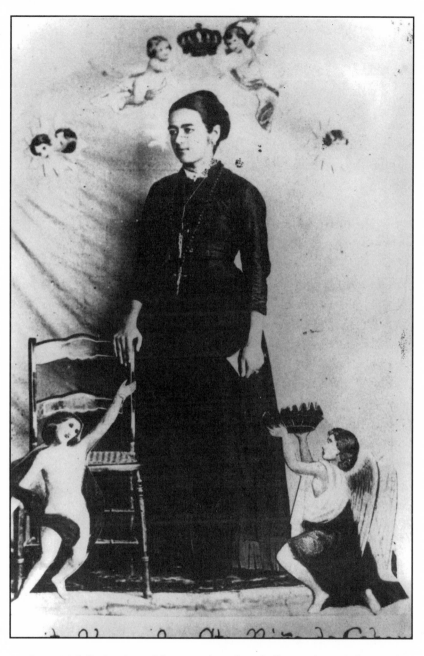

In 1896, believing it would protect them from bullets, Indian rebels carried this image of Teresa Urrea (note misspelling), "the Saint of Cabora," into battle against the Mexican government.
Photo courtesy Arizona Historical Society, neg. no. 1671.

most priests looked with tolerance upon Teresita's early healing activities, when a large percentage of the population of three states began to call her the Saint of Cabora, they began to impress on their congregations the difference between a healer and a saint. The status of sainthood, they explained, could only be conferred by the Sacred Congregation of Rites in Rome after a long and tedious procedure, and sainthood was rarely conferred during an individual's lifetime. As Teresita's fame increased, a few priests denounced her as a charlatan. Although Teresita found no fault with the church, she did occasionally criticize the priests, saying, "They often…take money from the poor under false pretenses."

An event that was to have significant political consequences occurred at Cabora on December 26, 1891. Twenty-eight heavily armed men arrived from the mountain village of Tomochic in western Chihuahua. It was known that Tomochic was in rebellion against the government and had already defeated two federal armies. The Tomochitecos, a fierce, religiously fanatical group of men with powerful physiques and thick black beards, had heard of Teresita's marvelous powers and had come to witness the cures for themselves. For four days they watched her healing—ultimately electing her as their village saint and placing a wooden image of her in the honored niche of their church.

The government moved with a great show of force to put down the rebellion at Tomochic. Two armies, each with about fifteen hundred men, converged on Tomochic. With less than a hundred men, Cruz Chavez, the leader of the Tomochitecos, attacked the approaching armies before they could unite. The battle cry of the Tomochitecos was "*Viva la Santa de Cabora.*" So great was their faith in Teresita they believed that she would resuscitate in three days each one who died in battle. The battered federal armies managed to consolidate and, after waiting for reinforcements, laid siege to the village, which they destroyed in ten days, after annihilating the entire population of Tomochic—about three hundred.

Subsequently, Tomochic became a symbol to the Mexican Revolution (1910–1920) just as the Alamo was a symbol to the Texas Revolution of 1836. Although the ferocious resistance of the Tomochitecos had been inspired by Teresita, she had done nothing to encourage it. A dozen other mountain villages, as well as the Mayos, invoking her help, took up arms against the government, but the federal forces moved quickly to suppress the uprisings.

No evidence has ever been found to prove that either Teresita or Don Tomas did anything to inspire these rebellions. However, it is known that delegations from Tomochic, from the Mayos, and from the Yaquis had sought Teresita's approval. Each had asked her, "Is it right for the government to take away our lands?" To each she had replied the following, which could have been construed by the rebellious groups as giving her approval: "God intended for you to have the lands, or he would not have given them to you."

Whatever the circumstances may have been, the government concluded that Teresita was a dangerous and subversive individual. Consequently, the governor of Sonora sent a battalion of soldiers to Cabora to arrest and conduct her to Guaymas, where she was held as a political prisoner for a time. Soon thereafter, the Yaquis began converging on Guaymas from their river villages and forts in the Bacatete Mountains—congregating by the thousands around her house of detention, which "looked onto a cattle yard and where she was eaten by mosquitoes." To avoid a confrontation, the governor sent Teresita back to Cabora. Then one day federal troops arrived at Cabora, placed Teresita and Don Tomas under arrest, and took them to Guaymas, where they were put on a heavily-guarded train and sent to Nogales. On May 19, 1892, they were taken across the border into the United States and told never to return to Mexico.

Teresita's fame had preceded her, and the citizens of Nogales, Arizona, turned out to welcome her and Don Tomas, who were provided with a furnished house. On July 5, the Mexican consul in Nogales reported to the Department of Foreign Relations in Mexico that Indians from Sonora and Arizona were flocking to her in large numbers.

Don Tomas's household in Nogales was smaller than it had been for years. For several weeks, there was only himself and his daughter. Then Gabriela arrived with a large entourage. The trip of four hundred miles had been made in wagons, escorted by fifty Yaqui and Mayo Indians. With her came Don Tomas's bookkeeper, his "Knight of the Stirrup" (his personal servant), and domestic servants. Doña Loreto stayed in Alamos, where Antonio, her oldest son, was put in charge of the four ranches.

After the birth of Gabriela's sixth child following her arrival, Don Tomas moved his household to El Bosque, several miles north of Nogales. This place became the mecca for pilgrims seeking cures from as far away as Sinaloa. However, not only the sick and crippled came but political refugees as well. Nogales and El Bosque became rendezvous locations for revolutionaries plotting the overthrow of the Díaz government; for their cause they recruited individuals from among the throngs of people streaming out of Mexico to see Teresita. It was evident that the revolutionists were anxious to exploit Teresita's influence over the Indians and the Mexican peons.

After the family had lived at El Bosque about three years, the people of Solomonville, in the upper Gila Valley in eastern Arizona, sent a delegation urging Don Tomas and Teresita to move to their town. Don Tomas, wishing to distance the family from conspiracies near the border, consented.

Eight months later, in June 1896, the family went to El Paso, Texas. This move was occasioned by journalist Lauro Aguirre, author of *La Santa de Cabora*, who had been expelled from Mexico for his liberal ideas. Aguirre settled in El Paso and started a Spanish-language newspaper, *El Progresista*, dedicated to the overthrow of the Díaz dictatorship and the establishment of a democratic government. Whatever arguments he used to persuade Don Tomas to move to the border city undoubtedly did not involve participation in the revolutionary movement since the family had been maintaining distance from it.

The Urreas rented a large brick house in the 400 block of Mesa Street, then the fashionable part of El Paso. News of the arrival of *La Santa* spread quickly among the Mexican population, and soon crowds from both sides of the Rio Grande began congregating in front of the Urrea house. Subsequently, the demands on Teresita became as great as at Cabora. Citizens of El Paso were so favorably impressed with her activities that they provided a large tent erected on an adjacent vacant lot, where individuals could wait to be healed. When on rare occasions Teresita went about the town, crowds followed her through the streets. She always responded, and although she charged nothing for her services, many grateful people left anonymous gifts.

On August 12, 1896, scarcely a month after the Urrea family had arrived in El Paso, the invasion of Mexico by the *Teresistas,* as the revolutionaries called themselves, began. Seventy Yaqui Indians shouting "*Viva Santa Teresa*" charged across the border at Nogales and captured the Mexican customs house. The same day the *Teresistas* captured and held for a brief time every customs house as far east as Ojinaga, across the

Rio Grande from Presidio, Texas. However, before the day ended, the *Teresistas* were forced to retreat. According to an article on the front page of the *New York Times,* May 13, 1896, seven men died. Each had on his person a newsprint photograph of Teresita.

The conspirators had hoped that the attacks would be the signal for general uprisings all over Mexico, resulting in the overthrow of the Diaz dictatorship. But the attempts failed, due to lack of effective leadership. Probably the only person who could have sparked such a movement was Teresita herself. Had she been politically inclined and given the revolution her support and leadership, the Mexican Revolution might have begun in 1896 rather than 1910. Thousands of Yaquis, Mayos, Papagos, and *mestizos* of northern Mexico would have rallied to the cause—the same groups who later followed Villa and Obregon into Mexico City.

However, Teresita steadfastly refused to become involved with the political affairs of Mexico. On September 11, 1896, she issued a statement in the *El Paso Herald:*

The press generally in these days has occupied itself with my humble person in terms unfavorable in the highest degree, since in a fashion most unjust—the fashion in the Republic of Mexico; they refer to me as participating in political matters; they connect me to the events that have happened in Nogales, Sonora, Coyame and Presidio del Norte, Chihuahua, where people have risen in arms against the government of Sr. General Don Porfirio Díaz.

I am not one who encourages such uprisings, nor one who in any way mixes up with them, and I protest once, and as many times as may be necessary, against the imputations of my enemies.

In the month of October of the past year, I went out from a point called El Bosque, sixteen miles from Nogales, Arizona, where I remained with my parents three years and three months, giving my attention exclusively to thousands of sick people who were constantly coming to that place from all over the world in search of my services. I arrived at Solomonville the last of October of the same year, and remained there seven months, or until June of the present year when I came to this city; that is to say, three months have I resided here, and all this time have I given to my numerous patients, to whom, notwithstanding that I gave them all my attentions, I was unable to fully attend; the smallest number

I have cared for in one day being one hundred and eighty, although generally the number was placed at two hundred.

I should note that the local authorities of each place where I have resided, in view of my entirely peaceful and orderly conduct, have been pleased to issue me credentials of very satisfactory character which may be seen by persons in this community having occasion to look at them. My neighbors generally in this hospitable town also can testify to my good conduct. Very honorable persons in this community have thought it worthwhile to offer me their kindly offices in defending me; and as for me, my conscience is at rest in that I have never committed any misdeed. I extend to those kind people my grateful acknowledgements.

I have noticed with much pain that the persons who have taken up arms in Mexican territory have invoked my name in aid of the schemes they are carrying through. But I repeat I am not one who authorizes or at the same time interferes with these proceedings. Decidedly I am a victim since in a most unjust way I have been expatriated from my country since May 19, 1892. It is now over four years, and this expatriation was announced to my father and myself through General Abraham Vandala and José Tiburcio Otero, as being ordered by the president of the republic, Don Porfirio Díaz, by telegraph. Without doubt the haste with which he acted was inspired of my enemies; but I ask, would it not have been more just in this case, if General Diaz, instead of ordering me expelled, had consented to order a judicial investigation before the authorities of my place of residence that the tribunal might judge whether or not I was guilty of wrong doing? Nothing was done beyond expelling me, but this was in such a way that I and my family were forced to hunt in a foreign country the guarantees which our own country denied us. Oh, that heaven may pardon this ingratitude of which I have been made the victim by the president of the Republic of Mexico, with whom I condole with all my heart for being misled.

In conclusion I will state that if in the future more uprisings follow in the Republic of Mexico, and as, even now, it has been said by my enemies that I am the kind of person to start these movements, I will say once more that I am taking no part in them. Am I to blame because my offending compatriots demand of the government justice for me? I think not, and appeal to the judgment of every sensible person.

Teresa Urrea
El Paso, Texas
September 8, 1896

Despite Teresita's statement to the contrary, the Díaz government considered her presence in El Paso dangerous to the peace of Mexico and repeatedly urged American authorities to remove her to the interior of the United States. Several attempts were made on her life, and although it is not known whether these were carried out by paid Mexican agents, Don Tomas resolved to take no further chances. He arranged to move his family to Clifton, Arizona, a mining town sufficiently isolated without being too remote from his properties in Sonora and Sinaloa.

Clifton was a copper mining town located in a narrow valley cut by the San Francisco River through a range of granite mountains. A railroad brought in coal for the smelter, hauled ore from the open pit to the furnaces, and carried away copper bars. The workers and the tradespeople who supplied their needs lived in the narrow valley for a distance of three or four miles. Don Tomas appraised the town and found two items exceedingly scarce, milk and firewood. Consequently, to augment his income from the ranches in Mexico and to keep from being bored, he established a dairy and a woodyard. For the wood business, he employed fifteen or twenty Mexicans and purchased from fifty to sixty donkeys. These scoured the almost barren mountainsides for miles around for scrubby juniper growth. Both the milk and wood ventures were profitable, and he subsequently built a large house for the family and several small ones for his retainers.

Of this period, one of Teresita's half-sisters said, "Those were happy days. Illustrious and educated people came from as far away as Mexico City and New York to Clifton to see Teresita. My father's household never knew how many people there would be to eat or sleep. Teresita was always the life of the place. She played the marimba and the guitar, and sang beautifully. I remember so well how she charmed everyone."

The move to Clifton marked a change in Teresita's ministrations. Because of the isolation of the place and the small population in the area, the demands on her were greatly reduced. The town physician, Dr. L. A. W. Burtch, became a frequent visitor at the Urrea home, where he observed her treatments. Although he did not understand how she did it, often he saw she was getting results with some of his own patients whom he had been unable to help—mostly chronic and traumatic cases that had not responded to orthodox medical treatment. Consequently, he began referring such cases to her, and a lasting friendship developed between the doctor and Teresita.

It was probably due to Dr. Burtch's influence that the wealthy members of the community—the bankers, lawyers, and the American and British mine owners—became interested in Teresita's healing abilities. One of the bankers, C. P. Rosencrans, had a son about six, who suffered from the paralyzing effects of some malady, probably polio, and Dr. Burtch had been unable to improve his condition. He recommended that Teresita be allowed to try. In three weeks the boy showed marked improvement, and the American population of Clifton was impressed.

In October 1899, a worker in one of the mines fell in love with Teresita. There was nothing unusual about a man falling in love with her, for many men, including the Mexican general who deported her, had done so. The unusual feature was that Teresita fell in love with him. She had always said she intended to marry sometime. In fact, before she left Cabora, she prophesied that she would marry and that her husband would be mean to her and try to kill her.

The worker's name was Guadalupe Rodriguez, and he was said to be a Yaqui. The half-sisters remembered him as "tall, fair, and handsome." However, Don Tomas did not approve of him and forbade him to come to the Urrea home. A confrontation between them ensued when on the morning of June 22, 1900, Don Tomas was sitting on the veranda of his house when Rodriguez appeared with a carbine. This he pointed at Don Tomas and demanded his approval to marry Teresita. When Don Tomas quietly told Rodriguez that he disapproved of him and his idea of marrying his daughter, Rodriguez stormed around for a while, then went away. However, he returned in an hour with a justice of the peace and demanded that he and Teresita be married there and then. Teresita appeared, and a tense, dramatic scene took place, with Teresita being forced to choose between the father she adored and the man she thought she loved. Eventually, with an anguished look at her father she walked to Rodriguez's side and told the justice of the peace that she was twenty-seven years old and it was her wish to marry this man. The ceremony took place, and Don Tomas was never the same again.

Then Teresita went with Rodriguez to his lodgings, but this highly sensitive, mysterious woman was too much for him. In a subsequent interview Teresita told what happened:

The next day…he acted strangely. He tore up some things of mine, packed some of my clothes in a bundle, put it over his shoulder, and said to me,

"Come with me." The people who saw him said for me not to go, but I followed him. He walked on the railroad track. I did not know where he wanted to go, but I would follow. He began to run. I ran, too. He had his gun and started to shoot. The people ran out and made me come back.

Rodriguez continued towards Metcalf, up the valley a few miles. There, several hundred Mexican workers had gathered who had heard of the wedding and were furious with him. He had married their "saint," and saints were not supposed to marry. The Mexicans overpowered Rodriguez, who by this time had exhausted all his cartridges, and the sheriff placed him under arrest. He was then taken back to Clifton and put in the jail, an old mine tunnel with bars over the opening. A few days later he was tried, found insane, and sent to an asylum. Teresita's marriage lasted less than a day.

Following the demise of her marriage, Teresita went back to her father's house. A few days later, Mrs. C. P. Rosencrans offered to take her to San Jose, California, where a friend of the Rosencranses, Mrs. A. C. Fessler, had a three-year-old daughter dangerously ill. Five medical doctors had not been able to help the child. Whether her decision was prompted by her compassion for the child, or her unfortunate marriage, or her rift with her father is not known, but Teresita agreed to go.

A publication called the *Copper Era* described her leave-taking. More than five hundred people gathered at the railroad station. As the train pulled out, the crowd was a sea of waving handkerchiefs; women were weeping, and men were misty-eyed.

In San Jose, either Teresita, or nature, or a combination of the two, effected a marked improvement in the Fessler girl. Newspapers such as the *San Francisco Examiner,* the *San Francisco Chronicle,* and the *Call* sent their most sensational reporters to interview Teresita with the result that many articles and numerous photographs appeared. The *Examiner* referred to her as "Jeanne d'Arc of the Indians: a saint in a shirt-waist and a sailor hat."

After this success some clever promoters, impressed by Teresita's news value, began to explore ways to exploit her healing. They proposed to form a medical company, which would be privately supported and make her talent available to people of the entire United States. They would pay her $10,000 for a five-year contract. Possibly influenced by the Rosencranses and Fesslers, or because she no longer wished to be dependent on Don Tomas, she signed the contract on condition that she would never have to charge any patient for her services. It was her understanding that this was a philanthropic venture financed by wealthy people. However, she overlooked the fact that nothing was in the contract that prohibited the medical company from charging for her services.

Subsequently, the medical company launched the "Curing Crusade" with much fanfare at the Metropolitan Hall in San Francisco. Free exhibitions were advertised, and people were invited to come on the stage and be cured. The *Chronicle* stated that a thousand people attended the first night and that Teresita, cast in a public exhibition role, was ill at ease. Apparently, the public exhibition was the "come on" for the medical company then secured a suite of offices with theatrical arrangements and decorations where Teresita was installed. Although she was never required to charge a fee, clients had to pay a large sum to get in the front door.

After a few months in San Francisco, in January 1901 the medical company moved to St. Louis for several months. Teresita, who had never achieved proficiency in English, wrote her friend and native of Chihuahua Mrs. Juana Van Order in Solomonville, Arizona, to send one of her children as an interpreter.

When Teresita's request came from St. Louis, John, the second son, was the only one free to go. John was bilingual and four or five years younger than Teresita. After arriving in St. Louis, John became her professional interpreter and subsequently her husband.

Interviewed while in St. Louis by the *St. Louis Post Dispatch*, Teresita said:

We are on a world tour to learn the source of my powers, if possible. Some claim they come direct from God. Others say they are the result of some…physical peculiarity. Still others contend I am the medium of another personage, presumably a spiritual one. I do not know. Theosophists say that some astral body is making itself manifest through me. Whatever it is, it came to me while I was in a trance. I have cured thousands and expect to cure thousands more. I shall go to Paris, to Oberammergau, to Jerusalem, to India and thence to Egypt. Perhaps somewhere I may find someone wise in such matters who can tell me the secret.

The medical company then moved on to New York. While there, news came that Don Tomas was seriously ill with typhoid. Teresita, who was in an advanced stage of pregnancy, was unable to return to Clifton. Don Tomas died on September 22, 1902. A few days later, Teresita's first child was born in New York.

Although Don Tomas never returned to Mexico, there is evidence that friends in Mexico tried to intercede with the government to pave the way for his return. This he refused to consider, giving as his reason that he could never forgive a government that had expelled as pure and noble and Christ-like a person as his daughter. Instead, he became an American citizen.

Little is known of Teresita's activities in New York other than the fact that the medical company, probably for publicity purposes, entered her in a beauty contest, which she won. According to her half-sisters, considerable space was given to this event in the New York newspapers with photographs of Teresita dressed in robes and wearing a regal crown.

A planned world tour by the medical company never took place, however. Instead, the company went to Los Angeles in December 1902, where it is said that Teresita's treatments were given with theatrical flourish and patients were charged to gain admittance to the clinic.

In the spring of 1904, Teresita became completely disillusioned with the medical company, although the payments cited in her contract had been kept. She was pregnant with her second child and wished to return to Clifton. Subsequently, she employed a lawyer, who found justifiable grounds for breaking the contract with the medical company. She arrived in Solomonville in time for the birth of her second daughter, June 29, 1904, at the home of Juana Van Order.

Teresita had saved a considerable sum of money during her three and a half years with the medical company. As a result, she was able to buy a lot in Clifton and erect a large, two-story house with eight rooms. Here, she told local reporters, she "hoped to nurse the sick to health and to heal the wounds of the injured."

Despite her attempts to start a new life, Teresita was a changed person after returning to Clifton. She was moody and introspective, and with the birth of her second child, she seems to have lost some of her curing powers.

On October 15, 1905, a great multitude of relatives and admirers gathered at Teresita's new house to celebrate her birthday. All went well until the end of the party, when she made a little speech. After thanking everyone for their thoughtfulness, she then remarked that this would be her last birthday, and as the guests left she told each one "good-bye." This caused members of the family to recall how she had often said she would die at the age of thirty-three—having associated her life with that of Christ.

In December, the San Francisco River flooded Clifton, overflowing its channel and sweeping away many houses along its valley. Teresita was in the cold rain and water for hours rescuing people and their possessions. As a result, she contracted a critical bronchial condition that put her in bed for days. Although she was able to be up part of the time, she had forebodings and talked about her funeral, which she said would be soon. She wanted to see her mother before she died and sent a telegram to Cayetana, who had for several years been living in Nogales, Sonora.

Three days after Cayetana arrived, Teresita said in the morning, "I will not live through this day." Still, in the afternoon she walked to the kitchen and drank a cup of tea with Cayetana and her half-sisters. She was almost gay and related some pleasant experiences, after which she said, "I think I will take a little rest." She returned to her bedroom followed by a retainer, who arranged the pillows so she was comfortably leaning against them. Then, with a smile still on her face, she peacefully died before the family could be called.

Dr. Burtch's records show she died of consumption, but the family and other Mexicans said that she had worn out her spirit in the service of her people.

BIBLIOGRAPHIC ESSAY

This article first appeared posthumously in *The Southern California Quarterly* 45, no. 3 (1963) and is reprinted here by permission of the Historical Society of Southern California. The editor of the *Quarterly* thanked the late William Curry Holden for assistance with its preparation. Holden authored a full-length treatment of Urrea's story, *Teresita* (Owings Mill, Md.: Stemmer House, 1978). A descendant of Urrea, Luis Alberto Urrea is writing a novel based on her incredible life. Her story was also depicted in the documentary film *Nobody's Girls,* which aired on PBS in 1995.

"Teresa Urrea, Her Life, As It Affected the Mexican-U.S. Frontier" by Richard and Gloria L. Rodriguez appeared in *Voices: Readings from El Grito, 1967–1973* (Berkeley, Calif.: Quinto Sol Publications, 1973). Now exceedingly rare, Lauro Aguirre's *La Santa de Cabora* first appeared in 1896, published by his El Paso newspaper *El Independiente.* A reprint appeared in 1902, issued by his El Paso newspaper *El Progresista.*

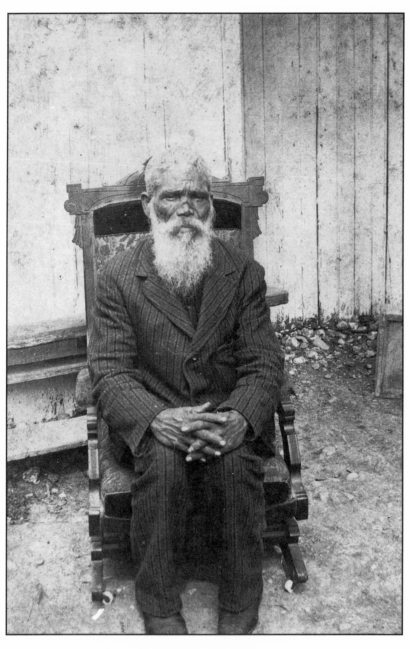

Faith healer Don Pedro Jaramillo, known as Don Pedrito, the Healer of Los Olmos, ministered to the people of southern Texas and northern Mexico from 1881 until his death in 1907.
Photo courtesy estate of James and Scottie Roddy Pirie, Institute of Texan Cultures, San Antonio, neg. no. 87-239.

Don Pedrito and Dr. Mud

GENE FOWLER

The reporter for the *San Antonio Daily Express* could hardly believe the scene. Hundreds of people, both "rich and poor," were lined up in a yard in "the Mexican quarter" of the city. Fancy carriages "attended by a coachman with livery" stood in the street beside primitive carts. "Silk dresses were crushed against the greasy blankets of the natives," reported the *Daily Express* in April 1894. "There was no distinction of class or race."

One by one the crowd inched forward. "Some are on crutches," noted the reporter, "some are bordered on either side by friends. Rheumatics, consumptives, paralytics, all are there. It is a wonderful and piteous sight." Reaching the front of the line, each stepped into the gaze of the famous *curandero* Don Pedro Jaramillo. Some had seen his photograph and recognized the long white beard and the gash on the bridge of his nose. And the eyes that seemed to look straight through a person and fill lost souls with hope.

The faith healer was visiting San Antonio from his home at Los Olmos Ranch near present-day Falfurrias in south Texas. In the Alamo City, Don Pedrito (1829–1907), as he was often called, set up in a shack behind the Grandjean estate on El Paso Street. At first, only the Mexican-American community called for Don Pedrito's unique prescriptions, but as news of the "wonderful cures" performed in such "mysterious ways" spread through the city, there gathered a cross section of the city's ailing.

According to the *Daily Express* account, an assistant, Blas Vela, obtained a patient's symptoms and then shouted the information to the deaf Don Pedrito, who then wrote out a prescription in Spanish. "Water, warm and cold, seems to be the chief medicine used by Don Pedrito," noted the paper. "It is used in the form of drinks and baths, taken at certain times and under certain conditions."

One sufferer was told to drink seven cups of water on Monday, Wednesday, and Friday mornings. Don Pedrito instructed another to drink one cup of warm water three times a week and to eat one pecan a day for twenty-two days. The healer gave "12 small Irish potatoes" to a woman whose daughter was "mentally deranged," and directed the mother to "put the fruit of the earth under the girl's pillow and have her eat one of them each morning."

City commissioner Bart Carruthers vouched for the faith healer's efficacy to the *Daily Express* reporter. Stricken with neuralgia on an 1892 trip to Rio Grande City, Carruthers had visited Don Pedrito at Los Olmos Ranch. The healer "told Mr. Carruthers that if he would pull three hairs out of his head, one from out of each temple and the third from the top of his head, he would be completely cured." As soon as he yanked the third strand, the commissioner told the press, "all the pain left."

Though one *Daily Express* report depicted a multicultural scene, another stated that Don Pedrito "will receive and prescribe for Americans during the forenoon each day and Mexicans, Negroes, and foreigners during the afternoon." At night he rode around town in a carriage to prescribe for sick persons unable to visit El Paso Street.

"He is an Aztec," proclaimed the paper. "The blood of that practically extinct but wonderful race flows in his veins. He does not know why he is chosen, but, impelled by something unaccountable, he is exercising a power that the Aztecs are said to have excelled in centuries ago."

But the healer refused to talk about himself, allowing only the puzzling revelation that "in 1897 he will be better known to the world." His assistant Vela told the press that Don Pedrito was born in Guadalajara in 1801, making him ninety-three years old. One statement said he was thrown from a horse (another said he was kicked in the face by a horse), causing the gash to his nose, as well as more severe injuries. "A strange woman appeared upon the scene to nurse him back to life," the *Daily Express* reported. In lieu of payment for her service, Vela said, she told Don Pedrito that he must devote the rest of his life to healing people "with the powers that he would find he now possessed."

The nature of those powers captivated the people of San Antonio. "The best physicians in the city have visited Don Pedrito and come away talking learnedly about hypnotism, mesmerism, and the faith cure," observed the *Daily Express*, "but the fact of the matter is they are dumbfounded and view with alarm the inroads already made into the ranks of their patients."

If so, the doctors breathed easier on April 24 when they read that Don Pedrito was leaving town on horseback. Vela and the healer had arrived in San Antonio on March 24. Between April 11, when Vela began keeping count, and April 24, when they prepared to leave, the *curandero* had received and prescribed for 11,583 people. Vela showed the reporter a stack of telegrams from as far away as New Orleans, sent by health-seekers who read of Don Pedrito in the *Daily Express*. The paper also noted that San Antonio businessmen had suggested to Don Pedrito that they manage him in a healing tour, but the "queer old man" declined all such proposals. "He averred that his powers were the gift of God and were to be received through the Holy Trinity for the good of mankind without cost."

Most accounts, including his tombstone, state that Don Pedro Jaramillo was born in Guadalajara in 1829 not 1801. South Texas folklorist Ruth Dodson, who collected Don Pedrito stories in the late 1920s and early 1930s, was told that he injured his nose (by unspecified means) while working as a laborer or shepherd in Mexico. In pain, wrote Dodson, "he went out into the woods to a pool of water. He lay down and buried his face in the mud at the edge." There he remained for three days, "treating himself with the mud."

The mud cured Don Pedrito, but the deep gash on his nose remained. Later, as he slept, "a voice awakened him and told him that he had received from God the gift of healing." The voice then instructed him to heal the owner of the ranch on which he worked. Prescribing the first thing that popped into his head, the novice healer instructed the man to bathe in lukewarm water for three successive days.

Don Pedrito moved north of the Rio Grande in 1881. Dodson noted that, before settling in south Texas, Don Pedrito had been jailed briefly in Mexico on a charge of being a *brujo*, or wizard. The *Daily Express* account infers that Don Pedrito exiled himself because the Mexican populace had become "terribly wrought up over his wonderful powers." In "Charismatic Medicine, Folk-Healing, and Folk-Sainthood," Octavio Ignacio Romano V described the charge as "practicing witchcraft" and stated that the *curandero* escaped from a Mexican jail.

South Texans also became "wrought up" over the humble servant of mankind. "Jaramillo was an enigma to his neighbors," stated the *Daily Express* in April 1894. "No one knew how he lived. He wandered throughout the country and was silent. He came and went from the ranches without vouchsafing a word. He treated the sick when they were brought to him, would accept no money or thanks. The natives feared and worshipped him."

Don Pedrito's south Texas practice lasted twenty-five years, until his death in 1907. Health-seekers traveled great distances and camped on the ranch. Given a hundred acres of land, the healer had it farmed and gave away the food to those in need. His *charro* hat and beard became familiar features in the region as Don Pedrito traveled by horse to visit the ailing at other ranches and communities, ranging as far as Laredo, Corpus Christi, and, as noted, San Antonio. Often when he returned to Los Olmos, as many as five hundred people awaited him. After 1893, they could come by train to a stop within a few miles of the ranch, then ride by hack to Los Olmos.

Don Pedrito healing stories collected by Dodson bear similarities to those chronicled in the 1894 *Daily Express*. Some of the unusual cures involved such actions as wearing tomatoes or garlic in one's shoes for a prescribed number of days. Others called for a certain number of sips of coffee or whiskey. A case of swollen neck was cured by rubbing olive oil on the feet. An 1893 victim of sunstroke was directed to go off by himself and bathe nine successive days. A señorita with heart trouble was instructed to drink a glass of river water five nights in a row. A woman who had suffered from epilepsy for thirty-eight years was reportedly cured by drinking one glass of water in her yard for nine consecutive nights, after gazing skyward and intoning, "In the name of God."

A few prescriptions appeared to use natural substances in more conventional ways—August flower for stomach trouble, *yerba del soldado* (soldier herb) for skin problems, and prickly pear poultices for dropsy. But in the great majority of cases, the faithful execution of the task resulted in the cure, or at least in the attitude adjustment.

Don Pedrito denied that he was a saint, but the healer's veneration continues to flourish long after his 1907 death. For decades, a Laredo entrepreneur marketed a line of herbal remedies under a Don Pedrito trademark, with the healer's picturesque visage printed on the packages. A spiritualist center in Monterey invoked his name for aid from the beyond. As the twentieth century begins to draw to a close, faith healers in Laredo and elsewhere in south Texas and Mexico prescribe remedies quite similar to Don Pedrito's, which are often applied in his name. And

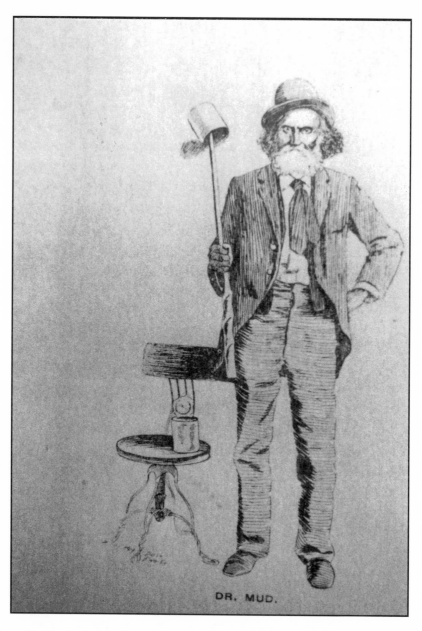

DR. MUD.

Dr. Mud, whose real name was Bazile Brown, administered his mud treatments to a multicultural clientele at the health resort of Sour Lake, Texas, from the 1880s until his death in 1903.
Portrait from an 1890s edition of the magazine *The Gulf Messenger*, courtesy W. T. Block, Nederland, Texas.

believers continue to make pilgrimages to his Los Olmos grave, while candles and figurines adorned with his image can still be found alongside traditional Catholic icons in shrines, homes, and shops far from the banks of the Rio Grande.

While the mystery of Don Pedrito was enthralling south Texans, visitors to the famed southeast Texas spa of Sour Lake often sought the healing ministrations of Dr. Mud. A former slave named Bazile Brown (18??–1903), the folk healer received his medical moniker from a Beaumont lawyer, who intended it not so much as a racial slur but as a reference to his treatments, in which he administered Sour Lake's medicinal muds.

Some tales of the source of Dr. Mud's healing abilities bear striking resemblances to some of Don Pedrito's. Thrown by a horse, one story says, Dr. Mud learned how to use the medicinal properties of the mineralized mud by treating his own injuries with it. All who wrote of visiting the spot agreed that Sour Lake had some very unusual mud.

Long a restorative site for Indians, the spring-fed lake sat atop a dome of salt and oil, which gave the water its curative qualities. The water's surface burped and boiled with the escape of natural gas, and most visitors noted the pungent presence of sulphur. In 1857, Frederick Law Olmsted described the "odd natural phenomenon" in *A Journey through Texas* as "having the properties of the Persian and Italian napthas." In 1882, A. W. Spaight noted in *The Resources, Soil, and Climate of Texas* that the lake and its adjoining wells were "in a constant state of ebullition, and the gases thrown off fill the air with odors of sulphuric acid gas, petroleum, bituminous tar, and other natural substances. Some of these wells are strongly alkaline, and floating on the surface of the water is a tarry film of the nature of crude petroleum." Crude oil cocktails, dispensed from pipes pushed a few inches into the ground and served by spa workers for twenty-five cents a glass, were a popular feature at the resort, located at the southern tip of a great woodlands known as the Big Thicket.

Shortly before his death in 1903, Bazile Brown told a reporter for the *Galveston Daily News* that he began his healing ministrations at Sour Lake in the early 1880s. Other stories said Brown had been born to an American Indian mother and a black father. Some believed him to be a native of Jamaica and attributed his healing powers to voodoo.

Beaumont journalist Ruth Garrison Scurlock, whose father had been an area Indian agent, collected tales from Dr. Mud's patients. They recalled the healer as tall and thin, with a "straggling" beard and a tall, stiff white hat like the one made famous by Grover Cleveland in his presidential campaign. In a long-tailed coat, with a crooked walking stick and trademark tin can full of medicinal pitch, Dr. Mud hobbled about the boggy, gas-burping spa prescribing various dirt treatments for his patients. He seemed to know instinctively which section of the lake held mud for certain maladies. Many women came to Dr. Mud for help with their complexions. The wizard was also a storyteller, especially popular with the children, who listened to him for hours.

Beaumont journalist Mrs. E. E. Edmondson wrote that "many a case of skin diseases yielded to the magic of his mud baths.… People, both white and black, came in wagons and on horseback to receive the treatment."

The patient sat on a wide board above a water trough, according to a description by Sour Lake historian L. I. Adams, Jr. "Old Bazile, 'Dr. Mud,' would select the mud that was to be used from several containers and after tasting each of the selections, he mixed and applied them to the man's body, rubbing vigorously on the affected areas." Often, the mineral-laden goo stung the patient's skin. When the health-seeker could no longer stand it, he dropped into the vat of water to remove the tarry balm.

"Being a man of God," Dr. Mud told the *Galveston Daily News* reporter, "I was directed by the Divine light how to use the mud, and everybody whom I treated was cured.… Sometimes parties who undertook to treat themselves made mistakes and aggravated the disease by applying the wrong kind of mud. I had to exercise great caution in this respect."

Careful as he was, however, the mud treatments often ruined the linen in the elegant Springs Hotel, built about the time the healer arrived in Sour Lake. At some point, hotel owners made him take his practice outside. Dr. Mud built two enclosures, for males and females, by the lake and called the clinic Ponce de Leon Springs.

In the 1890s, the San Antonio magazine *The Gulf Messenger* carried a tale related to Dr. Mud by an Indian named Chief Jim Black Cat. Long ago, said the chief, a hunting party camped at the spot that would become Sour Lake and made a fire to roast venison. Suddenly, the earth around them burst into flame and blazed wildly "until a broad but shallow hole was hollowed out in the ground." After a storm extinguished the fire, "the hole filled with water, full of medicinal properties sucked up from the earth, the benefit of which their medicine man was not slow to discover."

Dr. Mud told the *Galveston Daily News* reporter shortly before his death in 1903 that he knew that the heyday of his treasured medicine swamp was limited. The same geological conditions that had given Sour Lake its curative appeal caused its decline when an oil boom hit the area early in the century and the town was filled with seekers of black gold.

"Old Bazile" also knew his own days were numbered. "The Lord told me that the world might go against me, but it could do me no harm while he was with me," he remarked in the *Galveston Daily News*. "He tells me that the world, as well as my years, is drawing to a close, but no man knoweth the day or hour thereof. This is all plainly told in the Bible, if those who could read it only understand it. I can not read, but I know it is in the Bible because God tells me so. I am now over 80 years old but I know that God keeps me here for some good purpose. I have known Sour Lake about fifty years, but I only came here about twenty years ago by the command of God and will stay until he removes me...."

BIBLIOGRAPHIC ESSAY

Ruth Dodson's text on Don Pedrito appears in *The Healer of Los Olmos and Other Mexican Lore* (Dallas, Tex.: Southern Methodist University Press, 1951). "Don Pedrito—The Great Faith Healer" by Joan Draeger, published in *The Junior Historian* (March 1964) was helpful, as was "Texas's Own Saint—Don Pedrito Jaramillo" by William M. Hudson, in *Frontier Times* (May 1952). Additional information was found in *The Faith Healer of Los Olmos*, a booklet issued in 1972 by the Brooks County Historical Survey Committee, and in "Don Pedrito: Benefactor of Mankind" by Lennie E. Stubblefield in *The Cattleman* (August 1963). In addition to four newspaper articles from the *San Antonio Daily Express* of 1894 (April 8, 13, 22, 27), several recent articles were also helpful. *The Border: Life on the Line* by Douglas Kent Hall (New York: Abbeville Press, 1988) contains a recent photo of a life-size wooden statue/shrine of Don Pedrito in a Laredo residence. "Charismatic Medicine, Folk-Healing, and

Folk-Sainthood" by Octavio Ignacio Romano V appeared in *American Anthropologist* 67 (October 1965). Curiously, a negative and sarcastic view of his Alamo City visit appeared in the March 3, 1907, issue of the San Antonio magazine *The Passing Show*, which came out a few months before his death: "Some years ago an enterprising business man introduced into San Antonio a withered, aged and ignorant Mexican, one 'Don Pedrito,' and advertised him as a great healer. Within a few weeks the Don had one of the largest practices in the city, and among the best class of citizens. He effected many miraculous cures, all of which he could prove by testimonials. Unfortunately, his business relations became known and he then found himself called upon to discontinue his labor of love. Since then his 'cured' cases which have survived have suffered relapses."

Ruth Garrison Scurlock wrote about Dr. Mud in *Tales from the Big Thicket*, edited by Francis E. Abernethy (Austin: University of Texas Press, 1967). L. I. Adams, Jr., added some information in *Time and Shadows* (Waco, Tex.: Davis Brothers Publishers, 1971). The *Galveston Daily News* interview appeared on July 26, 1903. W. T. Block of Nederland, Texas, kindly provided a photo of a drawing of Dr. Mud, text from *The Gulf Messenger*, circa 1890s, and other information. A. W. Spaight's 1882 report, *The Resources, Soil, and Climate of Texas* (publisher unknown), is quoted in "A History of Hardin County," thesis by Mary Lou Proctor, University of Texas at Austin (1950). Frederick Law Olmsted recorded his Sour Lake visit in *A Journey through Texas* (New York: Dix, Edwards & Co., 1857). Mrs. E. E. Edmondson's material on Dr. Mud appeared in the *Beaumont Enterprise*, May 31, 1936. Other miscellaneous newspaper reports were found in the files of the Sam Houston Regional Library and Research Center in Liberty, Texas, and the Houston Public Library. One article from 1936 noted that Dr. Mud's photo resided in numerous Texas scrapbooks, but no photo of him has yet been located.

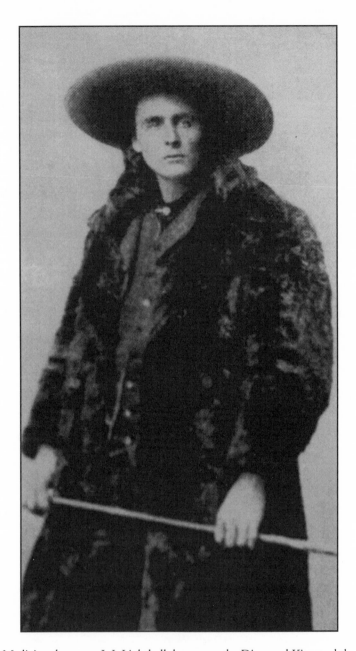

Medicine showman J. I. Lighthall, known as the Diamond King and the Great Indian Medicine Man, created a sensation wherever his troupe appeared. Fellow pitchman Nevada Ned Oliver saw "personality plus in the eagle eyes and handsome profile of Lighthall."
Photo courtesy the *Saturday Evening Post.*

The Diamond King

GENE FOWLER

It's made of barks, and oils, and leaves,
And seldom ever man deceives.
It never fails to satisfy,
And on it friends, you can rely.

It cures your aches, it cures your pains,
And everywhere an honor gains.
The way it cures it does beat all—
It's made and sold by J. LIGHTHALL.

San Antonio, Texas, December 1885. The Diamond King emerged from his tent and gazed about the encampment of his traveling medicine show. Brass band cowboys, midway Indians, minstrel singers, and other performers scurried from tent to tent, preparing for the grand procession to Military Plaza for the next show. Some groomed the medicine wagon's horses, recalled by Vic Daniels in *Frontier Times* as "dolled up in more gorgeous finery than any circus animals." Others polished the medicine-selling chariot, impressive with its ornaments of gleaming brass.

The showman checked his costume. Wardrobe was important when urging the public to buy medicines, and the Diamond King's outfits were varied and spectacular. He might have been wearing his ankle-length sealskin overcoat and large sealskin hat described by Fred Mosebach as "sparkling with diamonds arranged in designs of large stars." Or he might have been roostered-up in a red velvet suit recalled by Daniels as "tailored to perfection, of the old Colonial style, with all the buttons made with $5, $10, and $20 gold pieces," topped by a sombrero decorated with gold and silver, reportedly a gift from the president of Mexico. Whatever his attire, the healer's striking figure, noted Daniels, always blazed with "what appeared to have been almost a washtub of diamonds."

As the Diamond King climbed up to his "gaudy and highly attractive" wagon, he gazed across the street at the battle-scarred walls of the Alamo. From camp behind the old mission, the caravan made its way the short distance to Commerce Street, where it began the parade several blocks to Military Plaza. A crowd gathered behind the rolling spectacle, many drawn by the nickels that the Diamond King tossed onto the street and sidewalks.

At the time, San Antonio boasted the usual array of opera, theater, and variety shows, but the best entertainment in town was at Military Plaza's open-air bazaar, where the Diamond King's company joined an exotic scene perfectly suited for a medicine show. Barkers, hustlers, and pitchmen hawked jewelry, serapes, and herbs by flickering torchlight. Raven-haired "chili queens" sold spicy eats from portable stoves hauled by ox-drawn carts. Strolling troubadours vied for attention with shell-game operators and silver-tongued "professors." The greatest attraction, many believed, was the dramatic presence of Dr. J. I. Lighthall (1856–1886), also known as the Diamond King and the Great Indian Medicine Man of Peoria, Illinois.

After his troupe warmed up the audience with song and dance, the Diamond King stepped forward and offered to pull teeth free of charge. A line formed quickly, and, as Mosebach stated, Doc Lighthall was "busy as a butcher preparing a barbeque dinner for a firemen's picnic, hurling molars and incisors high into the air like shooting stars on a dark night as he extracted these from the capacious jaws of the victims with lightning rapidity. The patients were seated in front of a bass drum pounded with deafening effect while the band played 'Johnny Get Your Gun.'"

Then came the doctor's spellbinding health lecture and sales talk. "Everybody in the throng of a thousand or more hearers that crowded around his wagon," continued Mosebach, "was convinced that he was afflicted with one or more of the ailments cited and lost no time to produce 50 cents for the small size or $1 for the large size as he wormed his way up to the wagon to part with his money and receive in return a bottle containing a brown liquid that smelled like a mixture of turpentine and whiskey." Coins smaller than a quarter were thrown back into the crowd, "causing a scramble like chickens going after corn."

The Diamond King apparently arrived in Alamo City shortly before Christmas in 1885, after he had "astonished Dallas," as the *Dallas Mer-*

cury put it. Lighthall's presence in the Lone Star State had been noted by a crusading doctor on the Texas-Indian Territory border in his publication *Texas Quackery*, a statewide roundup of medical mavericks. "While this collection is in progress," wrote Dr. Alexander Wilson Acheson of Denison, "there is traveling through the state a person, styled the Diamond King; gorgeously arrayed, with different suits, and on all a wonderful display of diamonds; attended by a brass band and excellent singers; pulls teeth for nothing; also performs surgical operations free of charge. His main object is to sell medicine—or in other words—practice medicine. Money is what he is after. He says so, and acknowledges that the diamonds, brass band, gorgeous wagon, singing, and pie eating contests are mere accessories to draw the crowd."

Born in Tiskilwa, Bureau County, Illinois, in 1856, J. I. Lighthall's expected lifespan stretched into the decades of the "final closing" of the American frontier. An open horizon lay before him, a vast stage for self-invention. According to the romanticized sketch of his life in his 1882 book *The Indian Household Medicine Guide*, the future Diamond King left home at age eleven with a "youthful ambition to try his fortune in the west."

Reportedly, young Lighthall trekked to Kansas and Indian Territory, where his one-eighth Wyandot heritage helped him form "a warm attachment for the Indians." The medicine man claimed to have developed a keen interest in the "vegetable kingdom" at an early age, with a "natural gift for botany and the herbal kingdom." Thus, he was especially drawn to the "Indian doctors, from the fact that they were all the time gathering roots, barks, leaves, and flowers." He apprenticed with the native healers, according to the sketch, and assisted with their gathering of "Nature's remedies," impressed with "the fact that the Indian doctors never injured their patients with their innocent remedies, and that they soon recovered without aching bones or a salivated mouth." He then reasoned that "what was good for an Indian certainly was good for a white man," and that it was his duty to introduce "the Indian Herbal Theory" to civilization.

Lighthall claimed to have spent thirteen years gathering this knowledge, eventually wandering through Wyoming and other territories "until finally he reached Minnesota with a herd of Indian ponies, there falling in company with a celebrated physician by the name of Dr.

Neff." While on a "tour of digging ginseng," Neff encouraged his protégé to go into business. "Taking courage from this physician, he put his knowledge into effect, first by selling his Spanish Oil, or King of Pain, Blood Purifier, Dentrifice, and Indian Hair Tonic, afterwards treating all chronic diseases according to the Indian theory, by which he has cured thousands of cases, and still extends a medical hand of help to all sufferers who may have faith and confidence in God's remedies, that grow in our fields surrounding us, our gardens and our yards."

Though a Dr. Neff did later travel with the Diamond King troupe, another version states that Lighthall's Minnesota ginseng-digging introduced him to "the old original 'Indian doctor,' Doc McBride, as nervy a man as ever backed a bobtail flush." As the *Peoria Journal* told the story in Lighthall's obituary, "McBride was then on his last legs. Poker, whisky and women had brought him in poverty to the verge of the grave. Lighthall was shrewd enough to see that there was money in Doc McBride's business if he only took care of himself, and as he already had the long hair and cowboy garb, and wild western aspect generally, he was pretty well equipped for the enterprise. On June 11, 1877, he made his debut as a 'big medicine man' at Brownsville, Minnesota. His gross receipts for the first day were fifty cents. In another town on the next day he made $12, and he made money rapidly ever since."

Other sources indicate that Lighthall didn't break into the medical entertainment business until 1880, at age twenty-four. Dr. N. T. "Nevada Ned" Oliver, the Shakespeare of medicine show personalities, recorded an 1881 encounter with Lighthall in Jackson, Tennessee. As Oliver noted in a 1929 *Saturday Evening Post* memoir, the Lighthall performance was the "first Indian medicine pitch" that Oliver ever saw. Oliver wrote:

> He was among the first and certainly most famous of the longhairs and the buckskins. He called himself the Diamond King, wore a bucketfull [*sic*] of diamonds—some genuine—had a display of Indian curios, sold Herbs of Joy or some such title, and did an office-consultation business, carrying a graduate physician with him to escape the law against unlicensed medical practice.
>
> There was personality plus in the eagle eyes and handsome profile of Lighthall. All of our kind were prima donnas and Lighthall most of all. He resented our appearance. "I've got this burg sewed up in my pocket.

Try and work against me and see how far you get with your bean bags [a reference to the liver pads Oliver was then pitching]."

I suggested that there was room for both of us, that I take a corner well removed from his. When he refused, I took up the gauntlet. Two huskers, both first-rate artists, had come to town that day, playing the saloons. I added them to our show and opened on a good corner a block below Lighthall.

When we struck up, Lighthall's crowd began to drift. His was virtually a one-man show and an old story by then. The next evening he made his pitch on the corner across from us and his war whoops could be heard on the Hatchie River, twenty miles away. We stayed ten days. After the second night, Lighthall packed up his Herbs of Joy and retired until we had quit the field.

By the time actor George Roberts of Elmira, New York, joined the trail, the Diamond King's troupe had grown to eight men and two women. They lived in tents "on the fat of the land," the actor told the *Elmira Daily Advertiser*, and "nothing was wanted by any of them that was not supplied." Roberts recalled that Lighthall was "a great favorite with his assistants" and a great humanitarian. "On many occasions when poor people applied for medicine the bottle was handed to them wrapped in a $20 or $10 bill."

Most of the medicine was prepared in Peoria by Lighthall's mother and her third husband, Isaac Wright. From the town that inspired one of vaudeville's timeworn maxims, the elixir was shipped in barrels to the itinerant camp, where it was bottled and labeled.

Lighthall's tooth-jerking prowess was not only a great publicity-getter but a source of pride as well. Roberts said the Diamond King advertised widely his record of "fourteen teeth in nineteen seconds without pain" and ran challenges to other dental performers in the show business paper, the *New York Clipper*. Sometimes he would ask the patient if the procedure caused any pain. When the patient said no, Lighthall would turn to his assistants and roar, "What liars these people are!" as the bass drum pounded in the patient's ears.

On the road, the Diamond King told audiences that he owned the finest home in Illinois and that his garden paths were paved with human teeth.

Actor Roberts also recalled a web of romantic intrigue among the medicine show players. "Dr. Charles Lockwood, a member of the Lighthall party, the title being picked up, became enamored of Lighthall's wife, and his love having been reciprocated the pair fled from the camp, taking a splendid pair of horses and medicine wagon, and made good their escape, finally taking up residence in Binghamton, New York."

Lighthall's mother's second husband, a man named Johnson, worked as a detective for the medicine showman and kept order in the camp. Johnson "worked up the case" and traveled to Elmira, New York, with Lighthall, third husband Wright, and actor Roberts. The healing entertainers disguised themselves, reached Binghamton, and drew Lockwood out of town "by a clever ruse." The Diamond King "then went to the Lockwood residence, surprised his wife, 'Kit,' and ascertaining where the horses and wagon were, took possession of them and speedily drove across the Pennsylvania line, continuing until he joined the camp at Richmond, Indiana."

In San Antonio, the Diamond King had to compete with a varied cast of medical performers. Appearing during Lighthall's stand were the Yellowstone Kit show ("Top-Ha-Wah, Yellowstone Kit, Prof. Goodson and the Rubber Boy on the street tonight" announced the *San Antonio Daily Express*), a blind phrenologist and lecturer, a traveling physician from the Missouri State Museum of Anatomy, and Dr. Gardner, "the Wizard Oil Chief." The *Daily Express* reported that Dr. Gardner found the city's liberal policy on elixir-pitching was not without limitations when he was arrested and fined five dollars for obstructing a public street after refusing a marshal's order to "remove his exhibition from Military Plaza." A traveling doc from Boston, the "renowned Dr. Flowers," advertised his special "psychometric" powers of diagnosis in the *Daily Express*, treating a "multitude" of San Antonians at the Menger Hotel. Many of the psychometricized went down to the railroad tracks to marvel at the "magnificent special car" that enabled Flowers to establish "the largest medical practice in the world with branches in every state."

Despite the competition and the bad review from *Texas Quackery*, the people of San Antonio took the Diamond King to their hearts. Many were enthralled by the extravagant claims of his introduction in the *Daily Express*: "Tomorrow afternoon the Diamond King will pitch 40 tents at the corner of Houston and Nacogdoches Streets. The camp will remain several weeks and the public are cordially invited to visit and inspect the greatest Indian medicine company ever organized. Teeth will be extracted by the Diamond King daily free of charge. On Monday night he will appear on one of the plazas wearing $300,000 worth of diamonds, the largest collection in the possession of any one individual in the world."

From opening night the show was drawing crowds and receiving booster notices in the press. Sprinkled among the columns of local news, some of the reviews were not objective news reports, of course, but paid advertisements in disguise, a common journalistic practice of the day. On Christmas Eve, the *San Antonio Daily Times* notified the city that "the Diamond King, the great medical wonder of the nineteenth century, is doing extraordinary feats in his nightly cures of the afflicted on Military Plaza. He drew a very large crowd last night and all were satisfied that there is considerable virtue in his medicines." The paper's Christmas Eve edition published a jocular front-page tribute to the show's popularity in an advertisement for Erastus Reed's furniture store. "The Diamond King," announced the ad in large type, "Pulls teeth with imaginative pleasure to his victims. We sell Furniture with Actual Pleasure to our Customers."

An established hit, the medicine show landed in the papers' city pages almost daily:

We have seen many attractions in San Antonio, but none have drawn such crowds as the Diamond King.

He holds forth at his usual place tonight.

The Diamond King is a great character. He amuses the healthy, heals the sick and infirm, and creates happiness out of misery.

While it may be that he gets his share of the profits, he certainly gives a strong equivalent in curative agents.

The Diamond King has so popularized his remedies with the people that they are asked for everywhere. Hereafter they will be on sale by druggists. Meanwhile the Diamond King is still in the city and appears on the plaza morning, evening and night with a free concert, lecture and application of his remedies for the afflicted.

At the Diamond King's camp several physicians are employed to treat all diseases which cannot be relieved publicly. Blood disorders, as well as other ailments, are cured by the remedies to be found at his camp.

When the first snowstorm in twenty years hit San Antonio that January, pranksters filled the air with snowballs. "The Diamond King was a conspicuous target," reported the *Daily Express*, "as he and several of his staff passed, and the crowd made it warm for them until the Diamond sovereign's watch chain got broken in the melee, and then he and his cohorts sought a snowbank and retaliated with good effect, and were finally enabled to run the gauntlet."

A week later, on January 20, the *Daily Express* observed, "Dr. J. Lighthall, who succeeded to his 30th birthday yesterday, was handsomely complimented by his corps and the Spanish band. The gifts and tokens were rich, costly and appropriate, but he modestly refuses extended notice of them."

For the next few days the Diamond King was missing from the news as Yellowstone Kit, "drawing large audiences at the plaza," edged back into the limelight. On January 24, the *Daily Express* noted the showman's effect on the local economy. "Yellowstone Kit, having received an order from Guadalajara, Mexico, for three thousand of his liver pads, a preventive for smallpox and yellow fever, has employed 23 women day and night for the last two weeks sewing the herbs in sacks to be worn next to the body."

That same issue of the paper noted the cruelly ironic reason for Lighthall's absence from the plaza. "The Diamond King is now down with the smallpox, and a yellow flag is now flying from his camp yard." A minor epidemic of the disease had broken out in the city, and San Antonians assumed that the Diamond King was infected on the plaza by one of his patients.

Local physicians believed that his case was a mild one, but its severity was aggravated by Lighthall's continued drinking of ice water after the appearance of pustules. The Great Indian Medicine Man of Peoria, Illinois, died around sunset on January 25, 1886, in the shadows of the Alamo. Despite the fact that "he received untiring attention from his widow and aged mother," reported the *San Antonio Daily Times*, "all that medical skill could do in his behalf proved unavailing." He was buried in San Antonio three hours later. Though Vic Daniels later wrote that his "death was deeply mourned by almost the entire city," the *San Antonio Light* reported on January 27 that the Diamond King's survivors were "looked upon as pariahs in the community, and literally could find no place to lay their heads until Mayor Callaghan offered them a temporary refuge at his ranch." That same day's issue of the *San Antonio Daily Express* quoted Sam Maverick reporting that "the Diamond King outfit is not on Prospect Hill, but on six acres of land belonging to the city 200 yards southwest of the I.G.& N. depot." Lighthall's clothing, tent, and other personal effects were burned to prevent further contagion.

Editors picked up the wire story nationwide. Though the *Dallas Morning News* referred to Lighthall as a "distinguished medicinor," most panned the medicine showman in their brief obituaries. Sharing space with those reports, of course, were advertisements for patent remedies of equally debatable efficacy.

The *Chicago Tribune* noted the Diamond King's romantic turbulence in its terse obituary: "Dispatches from San Antonio, Tex., announce the death of Dr. J. I. Lighthall, the famous quack doctor of Peoria, Ill., from smallpox. The dispatches are wrong, however, in asserting that Lighthall leaves a wife. The fact is that two wives left Lighthall."

Back home in Peoria journalists argued in print over the controversial figure. A *Peoria Daily Transcript* reporter caught flak from his peers for writing that Lighthall "had a great future before him as a medicine man." The *Indianapolis Journal* offered an insightful, somewhat tolerant view of the late showman. "The death of Dr. Lighthall disposes of a very shrewd and money-making mountebank. He was anything but a fool, whatever else he may have been. He had enough force in his composition to hold his crowd of followers, and was a good enough judge of human nature to profit at its expense. He was a man that might have been dangerous had his inclinations tended in the direction of lawlessness. As it was, he was an expensive man to the poor wherever he went."

Estimates of the Diamond King's wealth varied as well. Most reports stated a figure of $50,000. Actor George Roberts believed the amount much higher, recalling that the show took in over $100,000 while he was along. The *Fort Worth Gazette* noted that Lighthall "claimed to be worth $1,000,000."

Many of the reports alluded to the great success of the showman's Texas tour. The *New York Tribune* added a dash of regional bias, smirking that Lighthall had suckered "Texas greenhorns" out of a fortune with his "quack nostrums."

Reminiscing in *Frontier Times* in 1931, San Antonio writer Vic Daniels recalled a variation on the story of the showman's demise. Daniels had been told that Lighthall contracted smallpox in Mexico on a medicine-selling tour. An epidemic broke out, and he "quit his business, went out among the people of all classes and administered to them, supplying his own medicines, furnishing hundreds of them food and other necessities, and all without cost." The president of Mexico was said to be so appreciative that he presented the Diamond King with a glittering custom sombrero. "The doctor himself was believed to be immune from smallpox," noted Daniels, and San Antonians were "dazed" by news of the medicine man's illness. Legends of Lighthall's generosity circulated through the medicine show grapevine, and one veteran recalled in 1942 that a monument was erected to him somewhere in Texas in recognition of his charity.

Some of the obituaries noted that the Diamond King's demise was hastened by his drinking of ice water. This, reported the *San Antonio Light*, "checked the progress of pustular formation so violently as to cause death." A few cited it as direct evidence of Lighthall's ignorance, but the text of his 1882 book *The Indian Household Medicine Guide* indicates a reasonable grasp of late nineteenth-century medical knowledge.

"We are fearfully and wonderfully made," he writes, concluding an essay on anatomy. "We are a greater mystery to ourselves than all our surroundings." Still, he maintains with Hippocrates that "all men ought to be acquainted with the medical art," and he discourses in "common English" on physiology, hygiene, digestion, and climate.

Introducing a lengthy section on the "Indian Materia Medica," which details the physical characteristics and medical applications of nearly one hundred plants, Lighthall explains that "medicine never cured anything. It is the natural tendency of a majority of diseases to get well within themselves," free from medical aid. "Medicine simply assists nature to remove the cause that obstructs her acting in a normal condition."

His description of goldenseal, also known as yellow root, compares favorably with the plant's description in more recent herbals—with a notable exception or two:

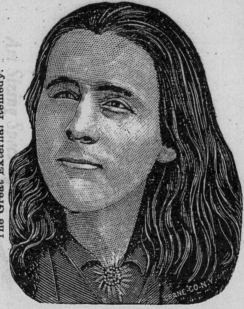

Advertisement for J. I. Lighthall's medicine company from *Gould's Peoria City Directory, 1885.*
Courtesy Peoria Public Library.

This root is one of the Indian's favorite remedies....It is admitted by all to be a fine tonic. It acts very gently on the liver, and as an alterative on the mucous membrane. It is a fine remedy in the treatment of dyspepsia and many other affections [sic] requiring a tonic treatment. It is a diuretic. When taken, it can, in a few hours, be smelled in the urine. It is a good blood purifier. To snuff the powder in small quantities in a great many cases will cure catarrh. Many a bad case of chronic diarrhea is said to have been cured by chewing the root as one would chew tobacco. It is splendid to take the powder and sprinkle it on an old cancer sore or ulcer. Take the powder and mix with water; this makes a fine gargle for a chronic sore throat, diptheria [sic], or any ulceration of the mucous membrane. It should be gargled some five or six times a day. The fluid extract, diluted one-half with water, and injected four times, is a certain cure for gonorrhea. It is unparalleled as an appetizer. The way it should be prepared so as to constitute a bitters for the stomach and the general system, is to take the root and cut it up fine and put in a quart bottle till it is half full, add one pint of alcohol or good whisky, and as much water, let it stand fourteen days, shake well once every day, and...you have a pure tincture ready for use. The dose is a tablespoonful or a common swallow before each meal. Crushed sarsaparilla, gentian root, and anise seed, will prove a great addition to it, acting as a blood purifier, appetizer, tonic, and alterative. If everybody, when first feeling bad, would commence taking this, they would seldom be obliged to suffer with fevers and bilious attacks. The Indian holds this as sacred to the welfare of his body as the farmer does paint for the protection and preservation of his house.

Many of the remedies combine two or more herbs. The Diamond King describes one brew that he used to build up his own brother when, after a lengthy fever, the brother was left "swarthy, weak, and melancholy," unable to take nourishment. "I recommended equal parts of the inner barks of poplar and dogwood and sarsaparilla root, cut up fine and put in a quart bottle until it was half full, then add whisky till full, and take a large tablespoonful, or a common swallow, before each meal." With this remedy, the medicine man's sibling put on fifteen pounds in a month. "It immediately increased his appetite, strengthened his nerves, and restored his complexion to its natural color."

Another preparation called for "Rattle Root, one part; Prickly Ash Bark, two parts; Poplar Bark, two parts; Sarsaparilla Root, two parts; Dogwood and Wild Cherry, one part. Fill a quart bottle one-half full of the above finely cut up, and add whisky till full. Dose, from a teaspoon-ful to a tablespoonful before meals. This will cure rheumatism, give an appetite, strengthen the nerves, and purify your blood."

Other remedies include blood root for cold relief, skullcap or mad-dog weed for neuralgic convulsion and spasmodic diseases, catnip berries for rheumatism, hops to help one sleep, and yellow dock for healthy skin. Surprisingly, the Diamond King ascribed to ginseng "no important or valuable medical properties." The herb was "gathered principally for the eastern trade" and made only "a very feeble tonic, fit for boys to chew." He praised quinine as "the king of anti-periodics and a deadly antagonist to malaria" but cautioned that "it should be handled with care as it often produces permanent injury, improperly given."

In a section on health care for horses, Lighthall included a story about one of his father's horses:

> It broke out of the stable in the night, and got into the cornfield and [ate] a hearty meal of green roasting ears, and the result was a fearful case of colic. The horse swelled almost to bursting. Father sent far and near for men that claimed to understand how to treat horses when sick. They gave soda, hot salt water, pepper, and a great many other things. The general prognosis was that the horse would die. I happened there at the eleventh hour. I gave the horse four ounces of aloes dissolved in a quart of warm water, adding to it one-half pint of good whisky, and a dollar bottle full of the King of Pain, or J. I. Lighthall's Spanish Oil, all at one dose. The horse soon quit groaning, and in eight hours had a free action from the bowels of undigested green corn, and then the horse got up and went to nipping grass and made a good recovery. I pronounce it a sure cure for colic. In case you cannot get the Spanish Oil, Perry Davis' Pain Killer will answer, giving two of the twenty-five cent bottles at one dose.

Opium, wrote the medicine man, "should not be used as much as it is" but should be taken "only in extreme cases, such as pain from cramps and neuralgia, wounds, mashed and broken bones, and then should be used in very light doses.... Mothers do a very foolish act when they give their babes Godfrey's Cordial, Bateman's Drops, or Paregoric. Children have been killed by their improper use."

That last sentence haunted the Diamond King's widow a few months after his death. She was carrying on with the show, her own jewel-studded image sparkling on handbills. In April, the Diamond Queen played Waxahachie, a small town south of Dallas, where her adopted daughter, four-year-old Sadie Lockwood, developed a cough. She gave the child a dose of remedy and then retired. During the night, reported the *Dallas Morning News,* the girl stood on a stool to reach the medicine, drank the whole bottle, and "lingered about thirty-six hours" before she died from an overdose of morphine.

There were, of course, hundreds of healing spielers like Lighthall roaming the country in the late 1800s. And whatever the ultimate judgment of his medical methods and sincerity, it's noteworthy that no less an authority than Dr. N. T. "Nevada Ned" Oliver credited the Diamond King with an important role in the creation of a western archetype—the long-haired, buckskinned Indian medicine pitchman.

Another source credits the medicine showman with a crucial influence on another milestone western event—the selling of barbed wire to Texas cattlemen. The report surfaced in 1948 in *Bet a Million! The Story of John W. Gates* by Lloyd Wendt and Herman Kogan, the biography of another son of Illinois. Nicknamed "Bet-a-million" for his impulsive gambling, wildcat financier Gates showed up in San Antonio as a young barbed wire salesman sometime between fall 1876 and spring 1878, according to most accounts. He soon found it easy to collect greenbacks from cowmen at the poker table but could not sell them on the newfangled wire. According to his biographers, Bet-a-million was sitting in the Hole-in-the-Wall bar facing Military Plaza, ruing his lack of sales, when he caught sight of the Diamond King holding forth with mesmeric salesmanship. Figuring what worked for snake oil would work for barbed wire, Gates determined to put on his own show. He threw up a corral in the plaza, ran a few dozen longhorns into it, and proved to the cattlemen that it would hold the animals without ripping their hides to shreds. As the story goes, the cattlemen found the show convincing and lined up to place their orders. Though it does not fit with the time lines of some versions of Lighthall's career or accounts of his style, and is probably a colorful invention of the authors, the story provides a nice mythological spin to the saga of the Diamond King. It anoints him, in effect, as the medicine showman who fenced the West.

BIBLIOGRAPHIC ESSAY

An earlier version of this chapter appeared in *True West* (March 1993). Original copies of J. I. Lighthall's 1882 book *The Indian Household Medicine Guide* are housed at the National Library of Medicine, Bethesda, Maryland, and other archives. Health Research (Box 70, Mokelumne Hill, California 95245) issued a staplebound, photocopied facsimile in 1966. Popular Library reprinted the book as *The Indian Folk Medicine Guide* in 1972. *Publisher's Weekly* (January 24, 1972) reviewed this now out-of-print edition as follows:

> Billed as "The Great Indian Medicine Man," the author of this fascinating book, first published in 1883 [*sic*], was clearly a believer in cure-alls and not the fast-talking con man we have come to equate with that type. Here are his recipes for natural remedies, using bark and wild plants, often mixed with equal parts of whiskey, and guaranteed to cure virtually every ailment of the human body. It is a delightful treatise and should be good fun for those who are into organic and natural foods for health—to sort out the real medicinal properties from the mystical and to relive the lovely, innocent days when Indian-white relationships were still hovering on the line between exploitation and genuine respect for traditions, old customs and wise ways.

Vic Daniels wrote about Lighthall in *Frontier Times* in November 1931. Fred Mosebach did the same in the *San Antonio Express*, November 3, 1933. The George Roberts story is from the *Elmira Daily Advertiser*, January 28, 1886. Thanks to Donald F. Woodard, Chemung County Historical Society, Elmira, New York. Adel Speiser covered Lighthall briefly in her thesis, "The Story of the Theatre in San Antonio," completed in 1948 at St. Mary's University in San Antonio, as did Midge Langendorff in her 1947 St. Mary's thesis, "The Medicine Man and Medical Fakeries." William P. Burt mentioned the Diamond King in "Backstage with a Medicine Show Fifty Years Ago" in *Colorado Mag-*

azine (July 1942). Dr. Alexander Wilson Acheson's views of the healing showman appear in *Texas Quackery* (Denison, Tex.: Murray's Steam Printing House, 1885); "Alagazam, the Story of Pitchmen High and Low" and "Med Show," Nevada Ned's (Dr. N. T. Oliver's) glorious two-part memoir appeared in the *Saturday Evening Post* (September 14 and October 19, 1929). The Bet-a-million Gates anecdote is in *Bet a Million! The Story of John W. Gates* by Lloyd Wendt and Herman Kogan (Indianapolis, Ind.: Bobbs-Merrill, 1948). Lighthall appears briefly (sometimes slightly inaccurately) in various San Antonio histories. A small amount of Lighthall material can be found in the "patent medicine" files of the Peoria Historical Society Collection, housed at Bradley University Library, Peoria, Illinois.

The Bradley University collection includes a flyer for Amole Diamond King Soap, "the late Dr. J. I. Lighthall's brand," which features the sparkling image of the diamond-encrusted medicine man and describes Peoria's Mexican Amole Soap Company's product as a skin-disease-healing vegetable soap, prepared for Amole in Las Cruces, New Mexico. "Teeth Extracted without Pain by the Celebrated Mrs. J. I. Lighthall," announced an ad for a performance in Seguin, Texas, which also promised stirring lectures by the "Little Big Medicine Man" W. Frank Wood, a long-haired fellow in fancy Indian outfit. The *San Antonio Light* reported that Mrs. Lighthall might move the medicine factory to San Antonio. No evidence of such a move has been found, but the Bradley University archive does include tax receipts and other items from south and north Texas sites where the show performed in the late 1890s.

Med-show veteran Violet McNeal wrote in her intriguing memoir *Four White Horses and a Brass Band* (Garden City, N.Y.: Doubleday, 1947) that medicine pitchwomen were rare. A report by a Fort Worth physician dated February 18, 1886 (in the *Texas Courier-Record of Medicine*, February 1886) included among the "quacks of the first water" then invading his town "one of genus petticoat who comes from Paris. Bedecked in a golden chariot, pulled by three steeds, she parades the streets and finally locates on Court square, she turns loose enough venom to scare old Father Time entirely out of Tarrant county. She pulls teeth, extracts jaw bones, and squeezes out wens enough to startle the natives; all 'without pain or price.' With music in the air she has perhaps slung more third-class anatomical filth around her chariot, than was ever slung around [by] anyone else."

One of the Diamond King's business cards is on display at the Frontier Times Museum in Bandera, Texas. The museum's founder, J. Marvin Hunter, wrote "The Diamond King: A Bunco of the Eighties" for his magazine *Frontier Times* (April–June 1953), a fanciful report that reveals the folkloric dimension of Lighthall's Texas legend. Sixty-seven years after his death in Alamo City, Hunter claimed that many folks still recalled the "furor" caused by this "singular individual" when he "electrified" San Antonio. "His Mexican sombrero was thickly powdered with immense gems," wrote Hunter, "all of the purest water, and as large as a hazelnut, it seemed." His coat, vest, and buttons were also "sparkling with diamonds." In Hunter's version, as in most others, he pulled teeth, sold Spanish Oil, and threw money to the crowds. "That man had San Antonio crazy. People fought for the privilege of being near his wagon. He swung the crowds as a man plays a horse, driving them from place to place, following his showers of money." But in Hunter's version, the Diamond King's death in Alamo City was a hoax; after the announcement of his passing, San Antonians felt such pity for the grieving widow of the man who had given away "every dollar that he possessed" that they raised and presented her with a small fortune. Then, wrote Hunter, "the Diamond King went from town to town, throwing away his money, selling his wonderful discovery, and dying of smallpox, and after each collection handed to his widow, he resurrected and again…he would quietly steal away."

Further proof of the fictitious nature of Hunter's story appears in the *New York Clipper* of March 16, 1889. Reprinted from the *Corsicana* (Texas) *Evening Times*, the report describes a memorial ceremony held in San Antonio three years after Lighthall's death:

Moving solemnly along Houston Street, and thence in the direction of the city cemetery, might have been seen, yesterday afternoon, a line of carriages headed by a brass band playing a funeral march. It was not a funeral, but in honor to the memory of one whose ashes have lain in the grave over two years. Dr. James I, Lighthall, who sold his medicine over the country by means of open air advertising concerts, and who was known far and wide as the "Diamond King," died in this city of smallpox on Jan. 25, 1886. To avert the spreading of the malady his remains were interred at night, and in the potter's field. His party, and his wife to whom he bequeathed a large fortune, subsequently left the city—and behind them remained the unmarked grave in the potter's field of the loving husband, and, in many respects, generous and good man. Thus it remained until Dr. Louis Turner came to San Antonio a few days ago. He was an intimate friend of Lighthall's, and learning of the latter's untimely death and unmarked grave, he immediately bought and had erected over the lonely mound a handsome monument, testifying his love and appreciation. Some of the employees of the local theatres who had worked for the deceased volunteered their services, and the procession was at this late day an honorable testimonial from friends in lieu of a funeral.

George Halleck Center and the Call of the Wild

ADRIENNE MAYOR AND MICHELE ANGEL

George Halleck Center (1855–1939) was a folk herbalist who sold patent medicines and practiced laying on of hands in southern Illinois from 1875 until the end of the Great Depression. As a young man, Center modeled his appearance on Wild Bill Hickok, eloped with a young Indian bride, and operated a medicine show. He worked nearly all his life in the coal mines and founded two local organizations based on his own brand of pro-labor, anti-Old Testament populist mysticism. An avid amateur naturalist, his taxidermy skills were much in demand, and his collection of one thousand birds' eggs ended up at the Southern Illinois University Museum. His writings and the memories of his children and grandchildren provide insights into the life and character of this self-taught healer, who defined himself in terms of the American West.

Center's parents, Andrew and Abigail Center, eloped in 1845 from New York to Ohio, where Center was born on February 25, 1855. When he was three years old, the family set out in a covered wagon for the new Oregon Territory. But when they crossed the Mississippi in 1858, wagon trains were halted at Cape Girardeau, in southeastern Missouri, due to Indian wars on the Platte River. Consequently, his father decided to buy a farm and two or three slaves about ten miles northwest of Cape Girardeau, near Jackson. There he raised oxen for wagon trains heading west, and Abigail worked as an herbal healer and midwife.

Late in life, Center reminisced about his Ozark childhood: "We lived in a log house with a huge fireplace, with a great flat rock for a hearth. On winter evenings when the chilly winds were raging through the hills, mother sat before the fire knitting. I, a boy of five, sat at her feet with her skirt drawn across my shoulders, as happy as a king on his throne." Abigail

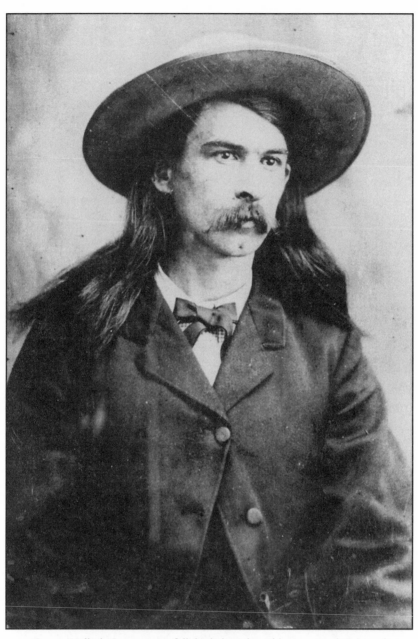

George Halleck Center was a folk herbalist who sold patent medicines and practiced laying on of hands in southern Illinois from 1875 until the end of the Depression. As a young man, Center modeled his appearance on Wild Bill Hickok, eloped with a young Indian bride, and operated a medicine show.

Photo circa 1880s, courtesy Adrienne Mayor and Michele Angel.

would sing sad songs at his request. Irish families fleeing the Great Potato Famine had settled in the area in the 1850s, and their song "Give Me Three Grains of Corn, Mother" about a starving boy "never failed to bring tears to [his] eyes," as Center recalled in the *Du Quoin Evening Call* in 1935. Then he would heat his mother's apron by the fire, wrap himself in it, and "dive into [his] trundle bed."

"My father and brothers worked in the timber, which enabled me to spend much of my time in the woods or roaming the banks of small streams," wrote Center in a 1915 notebook. These idyllic days "filled [his] young mind with a great and earnest love" for nature; reclining on a bed of moss, he would watch birds for hours. In a 1922 notebook, he recalled that his habit of capturing mice and lizards led his mother and sister to "make [him] turn [his] pockets inside out before they would let [him] in the house." His mother taught him about stars, insects, animals, and plants, and young Center helped her gather roots, leaves, and bark for her herbal remedies. Center's son Gerald Center stated in a 1972 letter that Abigail was an "herbologist of the first water." In a December 1995 interview, Center's daughter Lucinda Center Voight recalled Abigail's good education and "doctor books." Gerald, who became a professional pharmacist, still treasures the big iron mortar and pestle that George Center inherited from his mother Abigail.

When the Civil War broke out in 1861, Center's father Andrew exchanged the gold he had earned selling oxen for Confederate currency to help equip the Company A Missouri Artillery. "Naturally he went broke!" stated Gerald Center in a letter. Andrew served as an artillery captain with General Sterling Price, the last Confederate threat in the West, and he was a friend of "Swamp Fox" Thompson, the colorful Missourian who had been involved with the Pony Express and led Rebel guerrilla raids.

When Center was seven, his father was captured by Union cavalry and sent to Johnson's Island prison in Lake Erie, near Sandusky, Ohio. Andrew's two Yankee brothers back in Ohio had joined the Union Army in Sandusky, and according to family tradition they bribed guards to arrange Andrew's escape even though they disapproved of his politics. He returned to Missouri in late 1862 to continue fighting Yankees. In the turmoil of guerrilla violence that lasted well into the Reconstruction era, Abigail supported the family as a midwife and herbalist. When he had children of his own, Center used to thrill them with the hair-raising Rebel yell of his boyhood, and they loved to hear him sing "Give Me Three Grains of Corn, Mother."

After the Confederate defeat, Center's father established an amusement park in 1866 in Du Quoin, Illinois, a coal mining town about seventy miles southeast of St. Louis. The main attractions of Center's Garden, as it was called, were a primitive ferris wheel powered by two black men and fiddlers for dancing until the wee hours. There was a muddy swimming hole, and folks could buy cigars, beer, and soft ice cream. Some recalled that the park had an unsavory reputation. Center's father performed as a pugilist, and he may have booked Wild West attractions, such as sharpshooters, trick riders, Indians, and frontier personalities. To make ends meet, Abigail continued practicing midwifery and selling herbal remedies, and the children worked as well.

Center wrote in a 1915 notebook that his childhood ended "at the close of the civil war when [he] entered the coal mine as a trapper boy, at the age of eleven." Now he sat all day in utter darkness, ankle-deep in cold muck, operating the heavy ventilation doors for the coal cars. It was dangerous work: Center often recalled how many boys and men died in the mine shafts. In a 1922 notebook, he wrote, "I have spent fifty-six years of my life in the mines with hundreds of feet of earth over me, walled in on all sides with coal, which caused such intense darkness that Walpurgis night would have been twilight." However, young Center managed to continue his nature studies deep underground. Fantastic panoramas of branches and ferns were revealed by the miners' lamps in the coal tunnels, and he collected "thousands of coccle [sic] shells like gold" and the teeth of ancient sharks. When he asked the miners about these things, the "kindly but rough old men opened their think-boxes" and told him that these fossils had been "deposited in the mud when the world was young." Gazing at "picture galleries many millions of years older than the first pictures made by man," Center was awed by "great trees more than 100 feet tall and grasses, flowers, and ferns painted so thick one could not put a finger on the roof without touching a leaf."

"At the age of twenty," Center wrote in a 1915 notebook, "I married an excellent young lady who said she would share the joys, sorrows, and surprises of life with me." In 1875, he eloped (as his own parents had in 1845) with fourteen-year-old Josephine Eubanks (1861–1942), who promised to "stick to him like a burr." The two had met when Josephine was twelve; they eloped to Missouri to avoid trouble over the bride's age.

Josephine's father, Joel Eubanks (1839–1911), was the son of a young Cherokee woman from North Carolina known only as Nancy. According to family tradition, James Eubanks and his wife had rescued Nancy from the Trail of Tears in the hard winter of 1839. She lived and worked that winter at the Eubankses' house in southern Illinois; she was either already pregnant or became pregnant by James Eubanks. After the baby was born that spring, Nancy caught up with her people, leaving Joel with the Eubankses. The historical time frame, geography, and other details support the family tradition. Cherokees were officially ordered out of North Carolina in 1830–1835. In 1838, the U.S. Army began to drive the entire Cherokee Nation along the Trail of Tears to Oklahoma. Survivors of that tragic march did pass through southern Illinois in the winter of 1838–1839. Some thirteen thousand Indians camped on the banks of the Mississippi at Ware, unable to cross to Cape Girardeau due to ice floes, and two thousand died there of cold and starvation. The Eubankses, having left North Carolina themselves sometime between 1820 and 1830 (during the early campaign to remove the Indians), may have known or had blood ties to Cherokees. It is interesting that Nancy is a traditional Cherokee name.

Center taught his child bride to read and write and embarked on a concentrated program of educating himself. In "18 months I could read any book printed in English and through them I traveled the world over," Center stated in a 1915 notebook. His reading program included the Bible and classical texts such as Herodotus and Aristotle, as well as "Dr. Wood's Botany, Jourdans Animals with a Backbone, and Dr. Conges Key to Birds of North America." He began filling writing tablets with homely descriptions of the life cycles of caterpillars and the germination of seeds, marveling in a 1922 notebook over the incredible variety of life-forms from "microscopic moss" to giant "red woods of California." The nature notes are intermingled with notes on exotic cultures, from ancient Persia and Lake Titicaca in Peru to the Esquimaux and the Illinois mound-builders.

Center also wrote about Chicago sweatshops, "where factory girls get the enormous sum of 8 cents an hour." The girls' plight and his own years in the dismal mines started him on a lifelong crusade against "big shot" capitalists and organized religion's promises of "mansions in the sky instead of decent wages." Many of his notebooks contain diatribes against theologians who encourage superstition in order to help the wealthy oppress the "toiling masses." Notably, in his tablets of 1896–1938 he never wrote the word *men* without adding *and women*, and he railed against child labor, which "robs the young of the joy of childhood, destroys self-assertion, and poisons minds." He expressed pity for people who "had the misfortune to become criminals" because of unjust social conditions, and he actively supported the coal miners' bloody union movement. A 1915 essay titled "The Clergy and the Common Herd" begins: "As one skinned-shouldered horse can sympathize with another, I with much sympathy dedicate this book to all burden bearers, that have lived, are now living, or ever shall live."

After the Civil War, the exploits of daring outlaws and gunslingers of the western frontier captivated the public imagination. According to family members and photographs taken between 1875 and 1890, young Center modeled his appearance on Wild Bill Hickok. That story is especially plausible, since Hickok (1837–1876) of Troy Garden, Illinois, had driven oxen in Missouri during the Civil War and had ridden with General Price's Missouri Rebels as a Union spy. Center's father also had driven oxen and served with Price in Missouri; and he may have told young Center tales of Wild Bill, who had courted a part-Indian girl in Kansas in the late 1850s and whose quick-draw reputation began in Missouri in 1865. Hickok was a popular figure at local fairs, racetracks, and saloons around St. Louis and southern Illinois; it is also possible that he visited Center's amusement park in the late 1860s. His murder in Deadwood, South Dakota, in 1876, when Center was twenty-one, was highly publicized. It was about then that Center began to assume a western persona and sartorial style. He had several tintypes taken of himself; with his level gaze, long dark hair and mustache, wide-brimmed white hat, ribbon tie, checked shirt, and black frock coat buttoned at the top, Center bears a striking resemblance to popular engravings of Wild Bill.

Around that same time, Center determined to earn a living selling herbal nostrums, a decision that offered an escape from the grim coal mines. Poor people employed in mining camps were prime customers for patent medicines, and Center would have been familiar with special folk cures for coal miners' ills, such as asafetida and wild cherry bark.

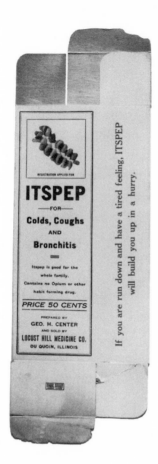

Package of George Halleck Center's medicine ITSPEP.

Photo courtesy Adrienne Mayor and Michele Angel.

IMPORTANT

The Great White Plague (Consumption.) — ι ... disease is the greatest enemy of man. Liveon, the ninety day consumption cure and Liveon Lung Discs—if ever equaled have never been excelled, for throat and lung diseases, especially consumption. We call your attention to the case of Tom Yancy, better known as "Preach," a young man of this city, whom the doctors said would not live thirty days. He gained twenty-four pounds in sixty days after using our remedies. Mr. Yancy is now with a show playing a very hard part, his lungs as good as new. Remember for Coughs, Colds, Asthma, Bronchitis and Consumption, Liveon and Liveon Lung Discs have no equal. For particulars write the company. Price 50c and $1.00.   LIVEON MEDICINE COMPANY,
519 N. Washington Boulevard.   DU QUOIN, ILLINOIS.

Advertising card for George Halleck Center's Liveon.
Photo courtesy Adrienne Mayor and Michele Angel.

Moreover, he already had a good supply of traditional remedies inherited from his mother's herbal practice, and he knew plant lore. This knowledge, along with his family's frontier and entertainment background, led Center to set up a traveling medicine show based in Du Quoin.

Medicine shows with Wild West and Indian themes began to draw crowds after the Civil War. The "medicine men" typically dressed in flamboyant western garb and wore long hair, and an Indian mystique surrounded their remedies. Son Gerald stated that Center's medicine wagon featured one or two "real Indians"; grandson John Mayor recalled stories about the show employing a "couple of white men dressed up like Indians" to drum up a crowd. Testimonials and advertising cards were distributed. Robert Voss, a grandson who was raised by George and Josephine Center, stated in a 1995 interview: "My grandpa told me about his medicine wagon. He said he had two Indians and that grandma wouldn't let them in her house." Also interviewed in 1995, John and Barbara Mayor recalled a photo of Center in western garb standing in the back of his wagon, with two men "with their hair parted down the middle and long braids, in Indian costumes" on either side of the lowered tailgate, and a blurry fourth figure (the photo was last seen in the 1940s; other relatives have denied its existence). Did Center's young wife Josephine participate, perhaps billed as an "Indian princess"? Other medicine shows featured "Indian princesses," and the family always referred to Josephine as the "granddaughter of an Indian princess."

Curios and exotic lizards and snakes were often displayed to draw customers. According to medicine show historian Brooks McNamara and others, venomous Gila monsters held a special attraction. As an amateur taxidermist, entymologist, and ornithologist, Center amassed an extensive collection of mounted stag beetles, butterflies, horseshoe crabs, birds, animals, and reptiles, including a Gila monster. By one report, Center had acquired the Gila monster alive and stuffed it when it died. But others claim that the lizard had been shot and brought to Center by the notorious local gangster-hero Charlie Birger, who ran bootleg liquor from Florida to St. Louis during Prohibition. Birger was hung before he could reclaim the mounted lizard. However, since no bullet holes mar the stuffed Gila monster (which is in our possession), the origin of this rare desert creature in Center's collection remains a mystery.

Center also set up an evolution display consisting of a human skull, a monkey skull, and mammal skulls of decreasing sizes. Robert Voss remembers sleeping in his grandfather's room crowded with ranks of staring owls, big rattlesnakes coiled to strike, giant long-necked snapping turtles, the legendary Gila monster, and the eerie display of skulls. The boy was warned never to open the closet door, because, as Voss stated in a December 1995 interview, his "grandpa kept a hoo-doo in there."

Some shows, like the Kickapoo Indian Medicine Company that traveled a nationwide circuit beginning in 1881, were huge operations with big budgets. Small outfits like Center's were known as "forty-milers" or "home guard" and performed in the vicinity of their hometowns. Center differed from the ordinary showmen and sellers of patent medicines, many of whom were con men hawking bogus cure-alls, in several significant ways. First, he had a strong family background of traditional herbal medicine and was widely read in biology and botany. Many patent medicine men had no medical knowledge and mixed batches of phony elixirs in hotel bathtubs or pitched nostrums for wholesalers who knew they were worthless. Second, Center believed in his remedies and formulated all his compounds himself, using many phytopharmaceuticals now known to be effective against the afflictions for which he prescribed them. Unlike fly-by-night quacks, he prescribed his remedies for his family and neighbors for more than fifty years and came to be regarded as "one of Du Quoin's most respected citizens," as the local *Evening Call* described him in 1939.

Oratorical discourses on the woes of humankind, the sorry state of the world, natural phenomena, and political and religious controversies were a common staple of independent medicine showmen. Center left a series of notebooks filled with fiery "lectures" on the exploitation of laborers by the wealthy; the current revolutions in Russia, Mexico, and Spain; the hypocrisy of elites since biblical times; and evolution and biology. The impassioned literary style and subjects of these notebooks suggest that they may have developed from oral disquisitions from his medicine wagon days. The most successful pitchmen always avoided sounding too slick, and in this vein every one of Center's highly rhetorical essays' opens with the disclaimer "I lay no claim to literary ability."

Center operated his medicine show between 1875, after he eloped with Josephine, and about 1880. It is unclear when or why he stopped going on the road with the medicine wagon. Perhaps the carnival aspect conflicted with his idealistic self-image; maybe he ran into legal trouble on the road; or possibly he decided to return to coal mining after the birth of his first child in 1880. Whatever the circumstances, after making his reputation with his medicine show, Center sold his patent medicines from his home and in drugstores for the rest of his life. He kept the dashing western look until the turn of the century; in photos taken around 1880 his locks just brush his shoulders, but by 1890 he wore his hair several inches longer. Daughter Lucinda Center Voight noted that he tucked his long hair under a cap when he worked in the mines.

After Center gave up the medicine show, he drove his wagon to Springfield, Illinois (about 150 miles), where he passed the exam for coal mine superintendent. He was prevented from taking the position, however, because of his support of the United Mine Workers Union (formed in 1890). But by 1896 he was assistant mine manager at the new Hallidayboro coal pit near Du Quoin. After work, he made medicines and continued his nature studies. He got special permission to construct a log house and plant a large garden in the woods instead of living in one of the coal company's shacks for miners. He and Josephine had nine children by then; two more were born in the log home he called Jack Oak Castle. Sarah Frances ("Frankie") Center Mayor recalled that when she was little, white and black families came to Jack Oak Castle on Sundays to buy her dad's medicine.

Building an old-fashioned log cabin in the woods in 1896 was a bit eccentric, perhaps a conscious effort by Center to recapitulate his happy childhood in Missouri before the Civil War, and certainly in keeping with his image as a frontier naturalist. In 1908, Center built a Sears Roebuck catalog house in Du Quoin, where he was manager of the Majestic and Jupiter mines and other Perry County collieries. In the lot next to the new house, he planted an orchard of native Illinois trees and medicinal plants.

Center's remedies and recipes are wide-ranging. Before the Food and Drug Act of 1906 regulated labeling and advertising of patent medicines, remedies were "often extravagantly described on boxes and labels . . . as 'sure cures' for a fantastic range of diseases," as Brooks McNamara put it in *Step Right Up*. Center's Liveon and Liveon Lung Discs, invented by him to treat "throat and lung diseases, especially The Great White

Plague" (tuberculosis), suggest that he definitely moved beyond his mother's traditional folk recipes. His use of an actor's testimonial reveals his sense of showmanship. The card advertising Liveon, "the ninety-day consumption cure," calls our "attention to the case of Tom Clancy, better known as 'Preach,'" a young local thespian who had been diagnosed as consumptive and given only thirty days to live. Liveon allowed him to recover in just sixty days, and Clancy went on to perform in a "show playing a very hard part, his lungs as good as new."

According to Gerald Center, his father had given Liveon (a tincture of rhubarb, glycerine, and alcohol) to two "white plague" sufferers and based his claims on their recovery. But either the claims or lack of a license got him in trouble. Center was summoned to court in Danville, Illinois, a wagon journey of over two hundred miles, where he paid a fine for practicing medicine without a license. After that he changed Liveon's recipe and toned down the claims, but the Liveon Medicine Company continued to bottle Liveon until 1917, when he sold the name and formula, reportedly to a large pharmaceutical company.

Twenty-eight of Center's recipes are preserved on signed handwritten (undated) cards (see Appendix B). Some of the recipes appear to be his mother Abigail's original formulas, such as the spring tonic "Ozark for the Blood" and "Center's Mother's Favorite Salve," calling for 4 ounces each of beef tallow, goose grease, beeswax, honey, brown vaseline, sweet oil, rosin, and 1 ounce of pure pork lard, to be "cooked slowly and well." Interviewed in December 1995, grandson John Dale Mayor recalled the "awful feel" of that greasy salve and the reek of plasters on his chest as a boy.

The herbal formulas contain botanicals whose properties have been shown to be beneficial for certain ailments. For example, "Center's Buchu Capsules for the Kidneys" contains equal amounts of buchu, an antibacterial effective against urinary tract inflammations, and queen of the meadow, a salicylate diuretic with positive actions on the kidney and bladder, as well as tansy, used in diabetes, and sassafras, a diuretic blood-cleansing agent. The strong painkilling properties of myrrh, the chief ingredient of Center's Liniment, were not isolated by chemists until 1996. The rhubarb extract in "Ozark for the Blood," "Liveon," "Lirusan," and other stomachics and liver tonics is an effective anti-inflammatory, analgesic, laxative, and digestive aid. The remedies for catarrh and bronchitis contain natural expectorants (asafetida, blood root), demulcents (black cherry bark, aloe), and licorice, which inhibits influenza A virus and bacteria in the respiratory tract—all ingredients favored by miner-herbalists attempting to treat coal-induced lung diseases.

Other plant extracts and substances are antimicrobials (cinnamon, sassafras), stimulants (aloe, blood root, capsicum), analgesics (laudanum, Hoffmann's anodyne, ether drops, sassafras, mandrake), cathartics (gamboge, aloe, rhubarb, colocynth, blue flag, pokeweed), anticarcinogens (clove, blood root), antispasmodics (asafedita, blackroot, ginger, fennel), and carminatives (cinnamon, fennel, caraway, gentian, peppermint). The zinc sulphate, acacia, salt, and rainwater of Center's eye and skin balms are still used for rashes and in ophthalmic preparations. In contrast to the phony tapeworm capsules of his day, Center's remedy contains kamala, a strong teniacide that does destroy tapeworms.

After the Civil War, opium was considered a wonder drug, and patent medicine manufacturers used opiates freely. Many soldiers had become addicted during the war, and hard economic conditions had led to widespread use of cocaine, morphine, and opium by the turn of the century. Until the Harrison Anti-Narcotic Act of 1914, laudanum was common in popular remedies. Center's "Cholera Prescription," for example, contained 2 ounces each of laudanum (opium), spirits of camphor, essence of peppermint, and Hoffmann's anodyne (or 1 ounce of sulphuric ether), 1 ounce ginger, and ½ ounce of capsicum (hot pepper). The dosage stated on the recipe card was "15 to 20 drops every 20 minutes until releived [sic]." This prescription would have had powerful antidiarrheal, antiemetic, antispasmodic, cholagogic, sedative, and carminative properties.

When Center sold Liveon in 1917, he changed the name of his company to the Locust Hill Medicine Company and replaced Liveon with ITSPEP "for colds, coughs, and bronchitis." The package states "registration applied for. Contains no Opium or other habit forming drug." Conservatively advertised as "harmless and pleasant to take," a batch of ITSPEP consisted of 10 pounds of brown sugar boiled with 3 quarts of apple vinegar, 3 quarts of wild cherry bark extract, and a small can of pure pine tar.

To grandson John Mayor, ITSPEP was bittersweet; his cousin Robert Voss says it tasted just like modern cough syrup. In son Gerald's mem-

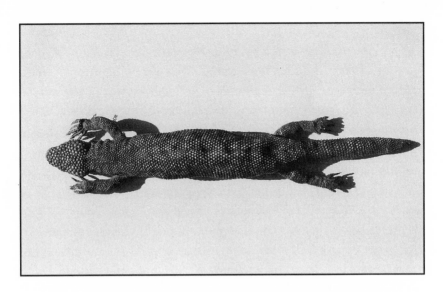

George Halleck Center displayed this stuffed Gila monster in the "evolution display" that accompanied his medicine show.
Photo courtesy Adrienne Mayor and Michele Angel.

ory, both Liveon and ITSPEP were redolent of turpentine. Center's
granddaughter Josephine Strauss preferred the "hickory smoke" flavor of
Liveon to the bland ITSPEP. She has vivid memories of the wonderful
fragrances in her grandfather's laboratory, a small building with a wood
stove in the alley behind the house. John Mayor recalls his grandmother
Josephine stirring big, boiling kettles, while Center filled gelatin capsules
with dry powdered herbs at his desk. Granddaughter GiGi Maxwell says
that great pots of medicine used to be set out in Center's front yard, until
the federal government forbade the sale of patent medicines outside of
drugstores. A local druggist, Arthur Angel, did the fine weighing of
grains and grams and provided imported substances. Lucinda Center
Voight recollected delivering bottles of her father's Liveon to Angel's
drugstore on her way to school, while her sister Frankie was an enthusiastic order taker around town.

In the medical profession's campaign to eliminate patent medicines
around the turn of the century, pharmacists were divided. Many druggists, like Angel, stocked patent medicines. In 1914, the United Mine
Workers local voted unanimously to demand that the coal mine bosses
carry Center's remedies in all their company stores. The vote was an

expression of gratitude for Center's support of a dismissed miner in 1913. The wording in the minutes from the United Mine Workers meeting of January 23, 1914—"He stood by the union through all this trouble and now depends on the sale of his medicines for a livelihood"—suggests that Center himself was fired or quit during the dispute.

Only two formulas, Liveon and the emetic, were fortified with alcohol. Center saw liquor as a cause of crime and impoverishment among mining families and supported the anti-saloon movement in Illinois between 1870 and 1920. In 1895, several years before Carrie Nation arrived in Du Quoin to "hatchetate" several of the town's thirty saloons, Center began taking in alcoholics and founded the Lords and Ladies of the Cross to instill "higher standards of citizenship and abstention from alcoholic drinks," as reported in the *Du Quoin Evening Call* in 1939. As an alternative to drinking, he supplied a reading room with books, games, and nature collections. Admission to the reading room was free, but there was a secret password for members: "Star, Cross, and Crown," indicated by silently pointing up, crossing one's arms, and touching one's temple.

Several of Center's notebooks contain lectures or readings for members. In them he castigates God for cruelty in the Old Testament, satirizes the story of Adam and Eve, and demands fair wages and justice for common men and women. In a 1995 interview, John Mayor recalled his grandfather thundering, "All babies are born with a clean slate!" and, "*My God* never made a Hell!"

Perhaps in reaction to coal companies' control of mining town preachers, Center also founded the National Law Association, to counter the "lies of the pulpit orators," which served to "keep the heel of the rich on the necks of the poor and ignorant," as he wrote in a notebook. Center engaged in debates with local leaders of the Holy Rollers, Baptists, Jews, and Catholics and concluded that "religion and politics have ever traveled hand in hand against the social welfare of the common people." In a letter to Rabbi Isserman, he appealed to "thinking men and women" disgusted by theological hypocrisy to "break down intolerance and outlaw war."

In the early 1920s, in recognition of his scientific taxidermy skills, the state of Illinois gave Center formal permission to shoot rare birds. People were always presenting him with dead or nearly dead creatures to be mounted. Center recalled how as a boy he had captured a big bullfrog and noticed its wide mouth and lack of ribs. While he was examining the frog, a whippoorwill perched nearby: "The spirit of investigation had taken possession of me, I wanted that whippoorwill! A hunter happened to come that way and by request shot the bird for me," he later wrote in a notebook. Amazed to find that the bird's small bill "opened a mouth as large as the frogs and that its legs were short and weak," Center was "compelled to ask why these things are so." He learned that a leaping frog would be "layed up" most of the time if it had ribs and a neck to break. Both creatures need big mouths to devour insects whole, but the whippoorwill eats on the wing and so has no need for powerful beak or legs. "According to Darwin," he wrote, "all creatures including humans must obey the laws of evolution and survival of the fittest."

After Center gave up the medicine wagon, his customers came to his house after work and on Sundays. At some point he also began to heal by laying on of hands. By 1900 his reputation began to draw even more people from near and far. Du Quoin was a segregated town; grandchildren recall that black patients came to their grandfather's back door. Most folks came to be cured of headaches, fevers, and warts, and they left with bottles and pills. John Mayor, who lived with his grandfather when he was about thirteen, remembered in a 1995 interview watching in fascination as Center rubbed his hands together and placed them on a young girl's warts. In a 1996 interview, GiGi Maxwell reported that her grandfather's "healing hands" were unable to dispel a stubborn wart on her knee; she was struck by his long fingernails, which he said he needed for taxidermy work. She also remembered that he politely declined requests for out-of-town house calls. To avoid trouble with the medical profession, Center did not charge for laying on of hands—although some people left cash. He never accepted money from the poor or patients who had come great distances.

Lucinda Center Voight recollected being healed as a child by her father's hands in the 1890s. He would rub his palms together vigorously, and the sensation of heat on her forehead or ankle was very noticeable. Robert Voss received the same treatment for childhood illnesses throughout the 1920s and recalls the warmth of Center's hands—in sharp contrast to the cold scissors Center would drop down his back to cure a bloody nose!

Center always kept a special white pebble in his pocket and pressed it to people's foreheads—to heal them or to read fortunes. Gerald Center says his father had found the smooth white stone deep in a coal shaft and was struck by its incongruous brilliance against the blackness. In letters and interviews, daughter Frankie and grandson Robert mentioned seeing Center use the pebble to heal "gullible people." In a 1995 interview, Lucinda recalled her father using the stone to tell the miners' fortunes—usually "they asked questions about their sweethearts." Center may also have done character readings; in one of his notebooks he remarks that when a man's fingernail covers most of the last joint of his little finger it indicates a "lazy womanizer."

Center's life was shaped by the opening and closing of the western frontier, and the social and economic strife in the period between the Civil War and the Great Depression. An eclectic autodidact with a strong sense of justice, he was attuned to the great ideas of his era, Darwinism, populism, the labor movement, pacifism, and socialism. As reported in the *Du Quoin Evening Call* in 1939, he was always skeptical of "preachers in business suits," and he "aligned himself with the forces that contrive for the better things in the community."

The contradictions of his life reflected the tensions of his day: His father had been a slave-owning Rebel, but Center deeply admired Abraham Lincoln. He became a mine manager yet remained fiercely sympathetic to laborers. He disdained traditional theology and "religious foolishness" but founded two religious groups. His youthful adventure as a medicine showman matured into a career as a compassionate healer, but he retained a flair for theatrical showmanship. He railed against superstition, yet he healed by laying on of hands and told fortunes with a magic pebble.

Indian wars had prevented Center's family from reaching the Oregon Territory when he was a child, and the aftermath of the Civil War consigned him to a life in the dreary coal mines; yet he kept his boyhood passion for nature and never shook off a sense of restless yearning. A card found among his recipes carries the wistful words, "All most everyone hears the call of the Wild. The love of God, home and country does not at all times prevent our hearing it."

"This beautiful world has been a playground for me," he wrote in a notebook in his eighties. "Every blade of grass, every leaf, and the bark of trees is the home of God's creatures, and to pry into the private lives of these creatures has ever interested me." His grandchildren used to joke that only one thing could make their grandfather run: a butterfly. According to all who knew him, Center carried on a lifelong romance with his wife ("Setch a woman!" he would often exclaim). At eighty-two he composed a love poem to Josephine, noting that the old tree where they used to bait their fishhooks in the early 1870s was still standing in 1937. A year or so later, Center fell ill (probably of heart failure). He died at home in Du Quoin in January 1939. In his last days, he refused to rest in bed. Preferring to sit in a chair, he told his children, "I'll be stretched out soon enough!"

BIBLIOGRAPHIC ESSAY

George Halleck Center's medicine company and recipes went to his wife Josephine after his death, who willed them to their daughter Frankie in 1942. Frankie attempted to reestablish her father's remedies under the name Golden Rule Medicine Company in the late 1950s, but her efforts to renew the old patents were unsuccessful, and the recipes came into the possession of her son John Mayor in 1969.

Center left eight notebooks, correspondence and other writings, twenty-eight herbal recipes, advertising and packaging materials, and nature specimens. Other original material includes family letters, photographs, and clippings from the *Du Quoin Evening Call* (much of this material has been donated to the Pearson Museum of Medical History, Springfield, Illinois).

This article would not have been possible without the genealogical research undertaken by Center's son Gerald Center (b. 1905) and his wife Florence of Pinehurst, North Carolina, who also shared photographs, advertising materials, and memories with us. We are grateful to Center's daughter Lucinda Center Voight (1890–1996) of Du Quoin, Illinois, for many conversations, memories, writings, photos, and newspaper clippings. Center's grandchildren Josephine Strauss (b. 1916) of Port Richey, Florida; Robert Voss (b. 1921) of Wauwatosa, Wisconsin; GiGi Maxwell (b. 1917) of Kewanee, Illinois; and John Dale Mayor (b. 1917) and his wife Barbara of Minneapolis, Minnesota, provided reminiscences, photographs, clippings, and writings by Center. The memories of Center's children Sarah Frances Center Mayor (1884–1969) and

Virgil Center (1888–1978) were also indispensable. It is not always possible to reconcile apparent contradictions between the recollections of Center's relatives and Center's own writings. We realize that some of the material included here is not accepted by all members of the family.

On early settlers in southeastern Missouri and southern Illinois, we consulted R. L. Gerlach's *Immigrants in the Ozarks* (Columbia: University of Missouri Press, 1976). Joseph G. Rosa's *The West of Wild Bill Hickok* (Norman: University of Oklahoma Press, 1982) describes the early career of Hickok and the images of the Wild West in the popular culture of Center's youth. In *Step Right Up* (University of Mississippi Press, Jackson, 1995), Brooks McNamara's lively history of medicine shows and showmen after the Civil War, we were able to trace similarities and points of departure for Center's healing career in the context of the rise and fall of patent medicines. Along with McNamara, John Parascandola, *Patent Medicines in Nineteenth-Century America* (*Caduceus: A Museum Quarterly for the Health Sciences*, Springfield: Southern Illinois University School of Medicine, 1987), and James M. Young, *The Toadstool Millionaires: A Social History of Patent Medicines in America Before Federal Regulation* (Princeton, N.J.: Princeton University Press, 1961), chart the medical profession's campaign against patent medicine makers and the resulting legislation.

George Korson's study of mining conditions, *Coal Dust on the Fiddle* (Philadelphia: University of Pennsylvania Press, 1943), contains valuable material on life in coal company towns; medical lore, religion, and politics among miners; and the temperance movement in southern Illinois. For the healing properties of traditional herbal remedies, we consulted *Herbal Drugs and Phytopharmaceuticals*, edited by Norman G. Bisset (London: CRC Press, [1989] 1994).

Indian John: Prairie Medicine Man

CHRISTINA C. Z. JENSEN

When Jacob John Derringer died at his home near the tiny community of Fact in Clay County, Kansas, word spread quickly across the prairie that the medicine man was himself finally gone. Widely known along the Kansas-Nebraska border as "Indian John," Derringer (1832–1924) was ninety-two years old at the time of his death. For forty years he had been a trusted herbalist and practitioner of folk medicine among the homesteaders in the area, credited by his neighbors with extraordinary diagnostic abilities and countless remarkable cures.

Derringer's career spanned the era of white settlement in the region, and he practiced his healing arts among these pioneering newcomers to the Great Plains. But his medicines were made from indigenous prairie plants, and his treatments were derived from Native American tradition. In Indian John's herbal remedies, the two cultures merged.

The medicine man first appeared on the Kansas frontier in the early 1880s, when he was already about fifty years old. A compelling personal appearance, obscure origins, and a mysterious background immediately provided him with a formidable mystique. Thale P. Skovgard described Derringer in his prime as a large but not fat man; over six feet tall and "straight as an arrow," with piercing eyes, a square jaw, and long hair.

Skovgard, at whose homestead Indian John sometimes produced his medicines, wrote in the *Greenleaf* (Kansas) *Sentinel* shortly after Derringer's death that "a most interesting story might have been written of his life and work, but with the traditional stoicism of the Indian and their disdain of praise, he steadfastly refused to give a connected narrative of his life." Instead, Derringer let a patchwork of fact and legend about his early life and training as a medicine man develop around him. It was a story as mysterious as one of the medicinal tonics he brewed.

Even whether Indian John was a Native American at all was, and remains today, a matter of considerable dispute. Cecil Rogers, who was an apprentice to Indian John in the herbalist's later years, wrote in an unpublished 1918 account of his teacher's life that Derringer "was born near Millesburg [Millersburg?] in Holmes County, Ohio, March 12, 1832. His parents were of American birth. His mother was a half Black-feet [*sic*] Indian and half French and his father was Pennsylvania Dutch." But Skovgard called his mother "a full blood Crow squaw," and the *Clay Center* (Kansas) *Dispatch* reported in 1955 that Derringer was "three-fourths Indian" and had Sioux ancestors. In its obituary of Indian John the *Greenleaf Sentinel* described him as a white child, born near Lawrence, Kansas.

As if Derringer's mixed ancestry weren't enough to explain his later interest in Native American herbal medicine, all accounts of his early life also include a version of his childhood abduction by Indians. Some say this happened near Rulo, Nebraska, or perhaps in his infancy near Lawrence, where his parents were murdered by the Sioux or Kiowa band that stole him. But according to other stories his capture occurred near Fort Laramie in Wyoming.

However, despite these discrepancies, all accounts agree that it was during his captivity that Derringer was first exposed to the healing techniques he practiced in later life. Some tales indicate that he was given an Indian foster mother or apprenticed to a medicine man of the tribe. These tutors recognized special powers in the boy. He was called "The Talking Crow" because of his unusually keen sight and hearing and an exceptional ability to catch the scent of men or game before they came into sight.

Yet the terms of his captivity were harsh. Cecil Rogers wrote that the Indians kept young Derringer under guard while an older companion "was given his free will, because the Indians knew that he would not leave without Young Jacob." After ten or perhaps twenty years, Derringer either escaped or was released. He subsequently served during the Civil War, possibly as a nurse. A commemorative quilt in the Clay County, Kansas, museum, embroidered with the names of local veterans, indicates that Derringer was a member of the 10th Ohio Cavalry. Later, he may have been a scout or an enlisted man under George Armstrong Custer during construction of the Union Pacific Railroad.

Cecil Rogers's version of Derringer's story states that he did not learn herbal medicine until after he was released from captivity by the Indians. "Then Jacob Derringer knowing what he had lost by not learning the medicine of the Indians…went to learn the medicine trade from a medicine man near Topeka, Kansas," the Rogers account explains. "There were four learning, with Jacob as one. It took them four years to learn it."

In such an apprenticeship, Derringer would have learned the ceremonial as well as the practical aspects of Native American herbal medicine. A traditional medicine man had to know the characteristics of prairie plants, their geographic distribution, and the appropriate times for gathering them, as well as specific techniques for preserving, preparing, and properly using them for medicinal purposes. In contrast to the surgical, technological approach to medicine that developed in white society in response to the terrible injuries of Civil War battlefields, Native American medicine emphasized harmony with the natural world. It was a broadly ecological view of the healing properties of plants with deep cultural and spiritual meaning for the Plains tribes, and Indian John adopted it wholeheartedly. Alma Nelson notes that, of the mainstream doctors and surgeons of his day, Derringer once remarked, "They are all butchers."

This, then, was the perspective Derringer brought to his herbal medical practice among the homesteaders in eastern Kansas and Nebraska. Sometime in the early 1880s, he settled first near Afton, a small community near the Washington-Marshall county line in northeastern Kansas. After a murder and a suicide among his friends there, and after a cyclone destroyed his house and blew all his possessions into the creek at a second home he established near a settlement called Swedesburg, Derringer finally bought the eighty acres near Fact in the extreme northeastern corner of Clay County that was his home until his death. It is said that this house had no floor because he claimed that without a floor a tornado could take his house but would at least leave his possessions behind.

The farm became Indian John's base of operation, but he worked from a number of outposts scattered across six counties on both sides of the Kansas-Nebraska state line. From his homestead near Fact and various outposts, Indian John traveled a regular circuit around his territory in northern Kansas and southern Nebraska. He rode a spring wagon

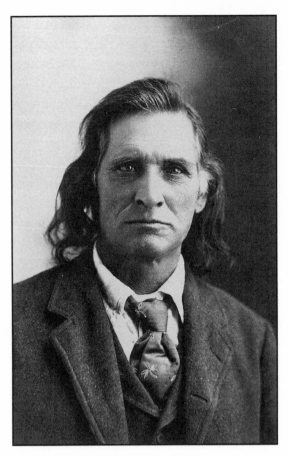

Known as Indian John, herbalist Jacob Derringer practiced folk medicine
along the Kansas-Nebraska border for forty years before his death in 1924.
Neighbors credited him with extraordinary diagnostic abilities and
countless remarkable cures.
Photo courtesy Washington County Historical Society of
Washington County, Kansas.

pulled by a two-horse team of paint ponies that was outfitted with a
square copper boiler tank from which his tonics were dispensed. The
tank had four separate compartments, each with a spigot.

All of Indian John's outposts housed both production of his medicines and storage of the plants he gathered. There, in large iron kettles,
he brewed a popular blood tonic made from the wild sage variety known
as white sage, or prairie sage, combined with vervain and crowfoot gold-
enrod. A kidney and liver medicine contained cottonwood bark, shoe-
string (leadplant), and sumac root. Colds and chest complaints were

treated with a brew of cocklebur, balsam, and burdock. Indian John used barks such as red willow, wild cherry, and slippery elm as well as the Plains' pervasive cottonwood. He gathered roots from herbs such as milkweed and ginger and the leafy parts of such plants as yarrow, cattail, mint, foxglove, feverweed, catnip, ginseng, napapoose, sunflower, and fennel. Evening primrose was the basis for one liniment he made, and he applied the leaves of the wild hemp plant to arrest female hemorrhaging. Moreover, he treated skin cancer with crushed sheep sorrel leaves and personally smoked mullein leaves as a substitute for tobacco.

Lobelia, or Indian tobacco, was Indian John's cure-all weed. Interestingly, the chemical lobeline, extracted from the blue lobelia flower, is today being studied for its potential use as a drug to help smokers quit without severe withdrawal symptoms. Other plants used by Indian John might merit similar reexamination. Although the vast stands of virgin prairie that once extended over the Great Plains have nearly vanished, the plants that filled these expanses remain scattered in pastures, yards, and along roads. One of these, prickly nightshade, or buffalobur, is described by the Kansas State Board of Agriculture's contemporary publication *Weeds of Kansas* as an "obnoxious weed hated by everyone because of its prickles, which are objectionable and uncomfortable to both livestock and humans." Today, the board recommends "good tillage methods" to destroy buffalobur, but the plant was found growing around Indian John's house after his death as though he had once attempted to cultivate it. Although the medicine man's use for the plant is not documented, it is possible that Indian John was aware of a beneficial property of the buffalobur plant that is no longer recognized.

The plant materials Indian John gathered were measured in bunches, which Cecil Rogers described as "a certain amount of herbs that a person can reach around with the thumb and forefinger." To make medicine in liquid form, each bunch was combined with a gallon of water and boiled for an hour and a half. Combinations of herbs required proportionally more water and longer simmering times. In one weekend alone, Indian John and an assistant could brew three hundred gallons of medicine.

Indian John made pills by boiling down one gallon of liquid to two-thirds of a pint and then mixing in two tablespoons of Epsom salts and about a third of a pint of flour. The stiff batter was allowed to cool for ten

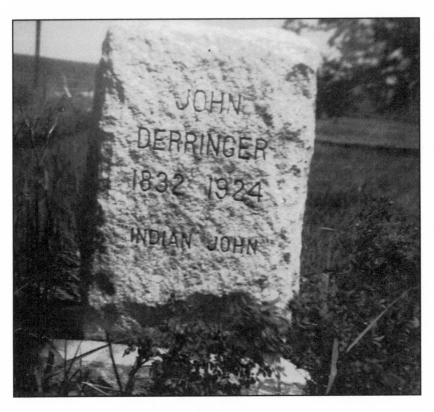

Indian John's grave.
Photo courtesy Christina C. Z. Jensen.

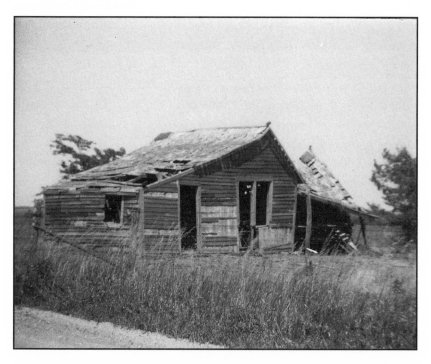

Indian John's cabin.
Photo courtesy Christina C. Z. Jensen.

or fifteen minutes before bits of it were rolled into pills the size of a kernel of corn.

The medicine man's formula for liniment, as noted by his apprentice Cecil Rogers, calls for half a gallon of king's cure-all leaves in one quart of hot water. The instructions conclude: "Remove from stove and pour in enough cold water so a person could work the leaves. Squeeze and work the leaves good and the liniment will be ready for use."

Apparently, Indian John practiced some veterinary medicine as well. Cecil Rogers's journal includes a nonherbal treatment for heaves and a cure for splints in horses that calls for alternating a hedge ball (osage orange) poultice with applications of liniment.

Indian John's treatments were affordable to his cash-poor neighbors. A gallon of his widely-used blood tonic cost fifty cents, and he was known to simply give his medicines away to those who could not pay. Moreover, because he maintained outposts and traveled his circuit throughout the sparsely settled region, Indian John was often available when and where a conventional physician was not. By curing, nursing, and comforting his isolated neighbors, Indian John helped many persist against the odds in homesteading the new and alien land.

Many stories have survived that testify to Indian John's ability to heal. One tale told about the medicine man involves a settler named Bine Fowler, who lived near Indian John's Rose Creek outpost in southern Nebraska. Fowler ventured out during a blizzard to care for his livestock, became disoriented, and could not find his way back to his dugout home. Although he survived by burrowing into a haystack until the storm passed, he suffered from a bad case of frostbite on his feet. For months he was unable to work. He and his family were preparing to abandon their homestead and move back East when Indian John arrived. The medicine man took roots from a sack, dug plants growing along a stream near the dugout, and boiled them together on the family's cookstove. He bathed Fowler's feet in this brew and applied an arrowroot salve. Then, after giving instructions to continue the treatment, the herbalist left. When Indian John returned to check on his patient three weeks later, Fowler was back to work.

Accidents were especially dreaded calamities among the settlers. One such disaster occurred near Belleville, Kansas. Early one morning, three freight wagons carrying stock salt were coming up a steep hill when the doubletree of the lead wagon broke. The driver was thrown, and the wagon rolled backwards into the second wagon, injuring the second driver as well when he jumped free and tried to block the wagon with a rock. Summoned to treat the injured, Indian John set bones in splints of bark and applied soothing lotions to ease the pain. By noon the freighters were on the road again.

Another time Indian John cared for the father and two children of a Republic County, Kansas, family, who were ill with a high fever. During the week Indian John spent nursing the family, he indicated a place near the homestead where a well could be dug to relieve the family and their neighbors of the burden of carrying water a full mile from the river to their high-land claims. When the father recovered and was able to explore the spot, he found the clean water Indian John had promised.

Indian John's dowsing ability and his uncanny gift for diagnosis were other examples of the unusual powers of perception that his Indian captors had recognized long before in the boy they called "The Talking Crow." Such capabilities refer to Indian John's highly developed physical senses and suggest that he had a kind of second sight. He was said to be able to see or smell a sickness, and once told one of his assistants that all common ailments and diseases have from one to five characteristic odors that a trained nose can easily identify. But smell was not the only sense Indian John relied on. He sometimes diagnosed through an intermediary—a friend or relative of a sick person who was not present—or simply by looking at a photograph.

In addition, he was supposedly able to identify the nature of an illness by examining an object from the sickroom. Once a piece of bedsheet was brought to him by a young Bohemian who did not speak English. Indian John immediately put the fabric in the stove and escorted the visitor out of the house, explaining that the cloth came from a room where there was smallpox. Later, his diagnosis proved to be correct.

On another occasion, reported by Joseph C. Jefferson, a man brought a handkerchief to Indian John, saying it had been on the chest of a sick child. But Indian John insisted that it had not been near the child. When the man then gave him a different handkerchief, Indian John smelled it and said, "Your little girl is well broken out with measles." The visitor was amazed and inquired how Indian John had known that the child was a girl. "In the same way I knew she had measles; and that first handkerchief came from a pocket where you carry rabbits," the medicine man replied.

A similar story is related about a young girl whose family was told by a Clay Center, Kansas, doctor that she had liver disease and nothing could be done. When Indian John happened by the family homestead on his circuit, the girl's father called him down from his wagon, saying "I'm sick and I need some help." Indian John replied, "You're not the one sick, and you know it. It's that little girl over there." He then looked closely at the child, told her that her liver was the problem, and promised, "I'll grow you a new one." The girl was cured in six months and is said to have lived to be at least seventy years old.

Commonsense psychology also seems to have played a part in Indian John's diagnoses and treatments. One young wife whose husband was always ailing tried to get him to consult the medicine man. He refused, but one day he laid aside a bandanna he had worn around his neck, and she took it to Indian John. After examining it longer than was customary, Indian John explained that her husband's problems would clear up if she herself applied the "no work, no eat" treatment. The cure must have worked, wrote Joseph C. Jefferson, because the woman developed a reputation as an excellent manager of a successful household.

On another occasion, a man came to Indian John's house to be treated for rheumatism. Although Indian John gave him the medicine he sought, for some reason the man sat down in a chair and refused to leave. Indian John grew tired of him after a few days and lit a small fire under the chair. His guest got up out of the chair quickly enough to indicate that his rheumatism was cured.

Although Indian John frequently took such a practical approach in his work, he was a profoundly spiritual man. His exceptional powers of perception were combined with an extensive knowledge of prairie plants unfamiliar to most settlers, and he honored equally both his Native American teachers' spiritual beliefs and traditional Christianity. He attended the Brethren Church in Washington, Kansas, for a time, but from around 1900 was a member of the Church of Jesus Christ of the Latter Day Saints. He shared the Missouri-based branch of the Mormon Church's opposition to polygamy. Because of his eclectic religious beliefs, Indian John was not always well understood by his neighbors. There was a rumor that he was involved in a secret spiritualist organization, and he was occasionally asked to perform witchcraft. However, he always refused, citing the Bible's prohibition against such practices.

In fact, the medicine man was so opposed to the occult that he refused to treat anyone he considered to be associated with it. One young woman traveled all the way from New York to be treated by Indian John, but he took one look at her and began to shout that she was possessed by the devil. As a result, she went away and washed off her big city makeup, and when she returned Indian John treated her complaint.

Folks who knew the prairie medicine man told researcher Gale Wollenberg that Indian John himself denied that his powers were supernatural and insisted, "I do not heal with divine power." However, he nevertheless made a subtle distinction and recognized the spiritual source of his healing art. Acquaintances told Wollenberg that Derringer said, "I prayed to God for powers to serve mankind." In a 1981 letter to the Marshall County Historical Society, Carl S. Nelson recalled Indian John saying, "My work is to make people well. It's God's gift to me."

Although Indian John never married, he had a great affection for children. Rogers wrote in his 1918 account, "Jacob Derringer has raised five boys and one girl [and] has given them each a farm." A doctor who later practiced at Palmer, Kansas, reportedly received financial support for his medical education from Derringer, despite the medicine man's scorn for the profession. Indian John also took in an orphan named Clarence Petry, who later joined a circus or a carnival. Moreover, Indian John's apprentices, like Cecil Rogers, who assisted him in gathering herbs and mixing medicines were often young people. The medicine man would pay them a few pennies for each pail or bundle of plants collected. Then every year all of these children and their families were invited to a large turkey and oyster stew dinner held around the date of the first frost at Indian John's homestead near Fact, Kansas. The mothers would bring food and help Indian John cook, and afterwards there would be a festive platform dance.

Children were also the beneficiaries of many of Indian John's cures. One year on the day before Christmas Eve a family named Carpenter from around Davenport, Nebraska, brought their son Bobbie down to Indian John's outpost at Rose Creek near the Kansas border. The boy had been kicked in the head by a horse two weeks earlier and had been completely unresponsive ever since. Indian John determined that the boy's senses functioned but that he had lost all memory. Consequently, the medicine man proposed a risky cure. He would give the boy a potion that would place him in a coma for twenty-four hours. After that the boy would gradually awaken; careful suggestions made during that time might cause his memory to return.

The parents agreed, and the treatment began. While they waited for the boy to awaken, Indian John and the mother arranged a seasonal scene around the child's bed—a small tree, pails of Christmas candy and peanuts, a crate of oranges, and even sleigh bells. Then, as the boy awoke, Indian John recited "The Night Before Christmas," and an assistant strummed "Silent Night" on his banjo as the mother called, "Bobbie! Bobbie! Wake up, it's Christmas Eve!" Slowly, the child stirred, turned to his mother, and asked where they were, for he recognized that he was not at home. She reassured him, and soon he joined the others in singing Christmas songs.

Although the healing of Bobbie Carpenter was especially dramatic, Indian John nursed many others through the common ailments and accidents of childhood. When Clara Koplin Meyerhoff of Linn, Kansas, was a child, children in her country school developed sores on their arms. Clara developed two red streaks running down her arm, which she later believed to be blood poisoning. To effect a cure, her mother applied Indian John's liniment.

Another dramatic case involved the treatment of a boy named Edward Nelson of Waterville, Kansas, for worms around 1890. A doctor had said that the child was too weak to survive treatment, but the medicine man's herbal therapy succeeded. Subsequently, Nelson grew up and married. A few years later his wife developed a large lump on her side, and the couple decided to consult Indian John before she underwent surgery. When they sat down with a group of ten others seeking treatment, Indian John exclaimed, "Hello, Eddie! There's nothing wrong with you that a little switch wouldn't cure." The Nelsons were astounded that Indian John had recognized his former patient after nearly thirty years—and even more amazed when Mrs. Nelson's tumor disappeared following treatment with Indian John's blood medicine, a cocklebur brew, and some salve.

Indian John's reputation continued to grow, and his practice matured with the steady settlement of the Kansas-Nebraska frontier. At the height of his career, he was sending medicines to clients in every state. In addition, he produced an advertising almanac containing some of his recipes. In his later years, he no longer rode his circuit; instead, his patients came to him. Scores of automobiles and large crowds filled his yard on Sunday afternoons.

Here he would gather about a dozen people in a semicircle before him. Without hearing symptoms or complaints but instead speaking to each in turn, he diagnosed their ailments and prescribed the appropriate herbal medicines. Witnesses on one such Sunday afternoon saw him rub an egg-sized tumor on a boy's arm and make it disappear.

Some who knew Indian John in his later years remember him as a filthy old man. Clara Meyerhoff recalls seeing rat droppings fall off a shelf above his stove into the kettle where the medicine man was brewing one of his tonics. It was for this reason that her parents, Fred and Katie Koplin, brewed their own medicine from one of Indian John's recipes. Alfred Lang of Green, Kansas, remembered him as having no teeth, "and when he smiled he reminded Alfred of the devil," writes Alfred and Clara's granddaughter, Susan Lang.

In spite of his remarkable record, Indian John never claimed to be able to cure all illnesses. On Christmas in 1923, he announced that his death would come from a cancer on his leg. The disease spread so that the healer himself gained a leprous appearance before his death August 27, 1924. He is buried in the rural Idylwild Cemetery a few miles from his homestead at Fact. A noncomformist in death as he was in life, Indian John's grave, rather than facing east as is traditional, faces west.

Indian John retained his faith in the land and its healing powers to the end, and his understanding of the medical potential of plant resources as treatments for seemingly incurable diseases was prophetic. "I cannot cure scarlet fever or diphtheria, but in some plant the Father-of-all has provided a cure for these scourges. The fountain of youth is all about; in back yards, pastures, fields, and along water courses," he insisted, as recalled in a letter by Rose Wiegert. Ironically, one of the places where native prairie plants are best preserved today is in undisturbed country cemeteries such as the one where Indian John now lies. Although his true identity and the exact nature of the healing arts he practiced are secrets gone with him to the grave, Derringer is still remembered in the part of northern Kansas and southern Nebraska where he gathered native prairie plants and brewed traditional medicines. His legacy is a belief in the land's power to heal and sustain—a belief that remains strong today among those who live and work along the prairie circuit Indian John once rode.

BIBLIOGRAPHIC ESSAY

Earlier versions of this article appeared in *True West* (March 1994), *Herb Quarterly* (Spring 1994), and *Nebraska Humanities* 3, no. 2 (1993).

Beginning with Thale P. Skovgard's account of Indian John's life that appeared in the *Greenleaf Sentinel* shortly after Derringer's death in 1924, the medicine man's story has been told by local historians throughout the Kansas-Nebraska border area where Indian John lived and worked. John C. Jefferson wrote a series of articles about him for the *Fairbury* (Nebraska) *Journal* in the 1950s; and features appeared in the 1980s in publications such as the *Salina Journal, Waterville Telegraph,* and *Marshall County News* in Kansas which reprinted Skovgard's account and collected numerous anecdotes about Indian John from old-timers who remembered him.

Alma Nelson's report, "Reputation of Indian Herb Healer Spread through the U.S." appeared in *The Advertiser* of Concordia, Kansas, October 13, 1987. Gale Wollenberg of Topeka, Kansas, author of *Indian John: Medicine Man to the Settlers* (Topeka: n.p., 1995), has compiled extensive information about Derringer. The historical societies in both Clay and Washington counties in Kansas have collections of materials about Indian John; librarians Cathy Haney and Jo Rippe have been most helpful.

While all of these sources have provided valuable information, my primary source and original inspiration for Indian John's story is Cecil Rogers's handwritten, 1918 journal account of his teacher's life. The journal was discovered at the time of Rogers's death in 1992 by his son, Wayne Rogers, and granddaughter Rose Wiegert of Fairbury, Nebraska. Rogers's descendants have graciously shared this unpublished manuscript with me so that Indian John's remarkable story might become more widely known.

The Weltmer Institute and Magnetic Healing in Nevada, Missouri

PATRICK BROPHY

On the eve of the French Revolution, Austrian physician Franz Anton Mesmer became the toast of Paris as the discoverer of "animal magnetism." By analogy to mineral magnetism, Mesmer theorized that a cosmic force, a "fluidum," sustains all life. Disease, he went on, was simply an imbalance in that force; right treatment was a "magnetic" transfusion, so to speak. That "one's batteries needed recharging" was no mere metaphor to Mesmer. Bitterly opposed by the medical establishment, Mesmer left little behind except his name immortalized in the word *mesmerism*—the hypnotic state induced in his treatments—and his ideas, which were still very much in the air in the nineteenth century. It was a time of conflict and interaction between science and religion, as well as of numerous intellectual movements, partly inspired by Mesmer, that sought to reconcile the two. Among the more famous movements were Spiritualism, New Thought, Theosophy, Unity, and Christian Science.

Another such movement flourished in Nevada, Missouri, from 1897 to 1930—the magnetic healing movement connected with the Weltmer Institute and related institutions. Although Nevadans still remember the Weltmer Institute today, few realize Weltmer was only the most successful of many magnetic healers, a half-page of which are listed in the 1900 city directory.

Sidney A. Weltmer (1858–1930) was born in Wooster, Ohio, though his birth is sometimes placed near Tipton, Missouri, where the family moved in 1858. His parents were well educated, his father having attended Heidelberg University, and his mother being the first woman to receive a degree from an Ohio college. Like many others, they fell on hard times due to the disruption of the Civil War. With frontier schools destroyed or dispersed, Weltmer would remain largely self-educated.

At age fourteen he met Dr. V. W. Brent of Tipton, who offered him the loan of his medical library. Such virtual apprenticeship was often the only preparation physicians received in that era. Weltmer's studies were interrupted, however, when he was stricken with tuberculosis. He later attributed his recovery to a study of the teachings of Christ. At age seventeen, he recalled in *The Healing Hand*, Weltmer "became interested in a little book entitled *How to Become a Mesmerist*," and over the next twenty years, he immersed himself in works on "what was then called Animal Magnetism."

At nineteen, Weltmer obtained a license to preach in the Southern Baptist Church, and within the next few years he was preaching in Sedalia churches, teaching at the local business college, and serving as Sedalia's city librarian. One Sunday he startled a congregation by telling them of his interest in healing; walking out before the service was ended, he declared that he would not return until he could do what Jesus had done in his healing miracles.

The aspiring healer formed a partnership with business manager J. H. Kelly and took to the road. In February 1897, the pair visited Nevada, where so many patients sought Weltmer's ministrations that he decided to make the town the home of a permanent institute of healing. His brother John and eldest son Ernest joined him, and within two years the concern had expanded into the seventeen-room house, built in 1886 by railroad contractor Frank P. Anderson (now a funeral home), dubbed the "Infirmary," with the "Business Department" next door in the former William H. Robinson house.

Weltmer advertised heavily, across the nation and abroad. By 1906, according to Warren C. Lovinger, Jr., M.D., the institution employed "seventeen healers, several assistant healers, a physician (for diagnosing organic disease)," and over a hundred stenographers and typists to handle correspondence. In 1901, the deluge of Weltmer mail compelled the federal government to raise the Nevada post office to first-class status. Weltmer was treating as many as 400 patients a day and advising up to 150,000 a year by mail. Nevadans told stories of employees carrying bushel baskets of cash to the bank. The *Nevada Daily Mail* put the institute's daily receipts at $3,600. The Missouri-Kansas-Texas (Katy) Railroad ran special coaches and Pullman cars from St. Louis, met by the institute's jitney. Boardinghouses to serve Weltmer outpatients became

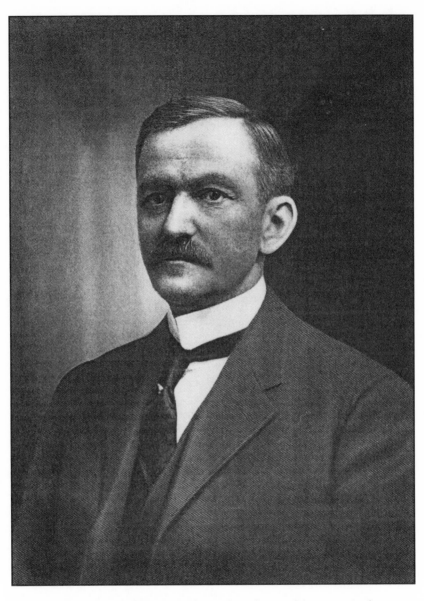

Magnetic healer Sidney A. Weltmer drew thousands to tiny Nevada,
Missouri, at the turn of the century
Courtesy Bushwhacker Museum, Nevada, Missouri.

the local growth industry. Notable patients and curious visitors included President and Mrs. McKinley, Harry Houdini, Luther Burbank, and John Philip Sousa with full band. Doubtless, the Sousa outfit played a local composer's "Weltmer March."

"Just now the eyes of the sick and afflicted in all parts of the world are turned hopefully toward Nevada," reported the *St. Louis Republic* on June 18, 1899, "whence reports of remarkable cures, effected through the system of magnetic healing, taught and practised by Professor S. A. Weltmer, are emanating daily." "At the hotels, in the streets, on the square—no matter where one goes in Nevada, he hears as the principal topic of conversation about Weltmer and his method of healing."

As the paper went on to note, Weltmer did not only practice magnetic healing but also taught it to others by correspondence course. In addition, the institute published numerous magazines and books, including one that seemed to underscore the economic advantages of the method, entitled *How to Make Magnetic Healing Pay.* However, success encouraged imitation; almost overnight, Nevada went "magnetic" mad.

"These institutions are very numerous in this city," grumbled the Reverend Dr. C. M. Bishop of the Centenary Methodist Church to a reporter from the *Nevada Evening Post.* "At the head of some of them are men who, a few weeks or months ago, were barbers or butchers or blacksmiths or loafers, and some women who were of notoriously bad character, who, after a ten day 'course' in magnetic healing, have become full-fledged 'professors.'"

The local debate about magnetic healing institutions continued among both secular and religious factions. Dr. Preston W. Pope turned out a booklet entitled *The Expose of Weltmerism: Magnetic Healing Demagnetized,* while Dr. E . L. Priest addressed a meeting of the Missouri State Medical Association at Sedalia on the subject of "Empiricism in Missouri and How to Suppress It." The churches staunchly opposed the philosophy of the institutions in a brochure, *The Ministerial Alliance vs. Magnetic Healing.*

"The lines have been drawn in our city," the ministers declared in the brochure. While the Commercial Club, a business group, had gone on record endorsing Weltmerism as a boon to the town, the clergy found it "subversive of the fundamental and vital principles of the Christian faith."

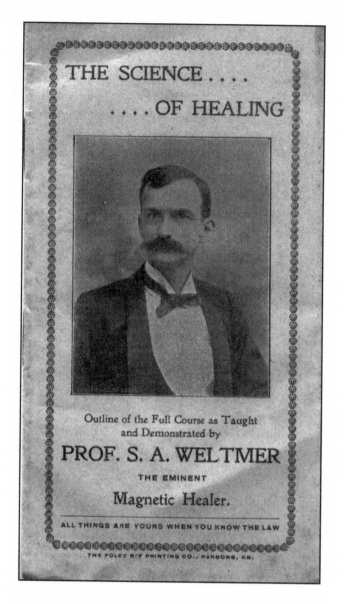

THE SCIENCE....

....OF HEALING

Outline of the Full Course as Taught
and Demonstrated by

PROF. S. A. WELTMER

THE EMINENT

Magnetic Healer.

ALL THINGS ARE YOURS WHEN YOU KNOW THE LAW

THE FOLEY R'Y PRINTING CO., PARSONS, KS.

Thousands of people sent for Sidney A. Weltmer's mail-order
lessons in magnetic healing.
Courtesy Gene Fowler.

Oddly, Weltmer appears to have ignored the physicians but defended the institute against the accusations of the ministers. In 1900, he and his business manager Kelly filed a lawsuit for "libel and slander" against Dr. Bishop and the *Methodist Advocate* magazine, in whose pages the divine had branded Weltmerism "a fraud and humbug," "an ignorant mixture of Negro voodoo and Christian Science," repeating charges first made from the pulpit. He hinted darkly at "lots" and even "cords" of bodies sneaked out of the magnetic healers' premises in the dead of night.

Since most residents of Nevada were partisan, for the trial venue was changed to the nearby town of Butler. There a new courthouse was under construction, so court convened in an inn—conveniently near a barroom, where trial participants seem to have passed much of their time. Before long, rumors began to circulate that Weltmer was buying the jury's drinks, and a sensation resulted when it came out that, in truth, the teetotal Methodist magazine had been doing so with secret funds.

As a result, on the stand the ministers' allegations were hastily curtailed. The trial transcript made juicy newspaper fare—ironically bracketed by magnetic healers' blue-sky ads. Found guilty, Bishop was ordered to pay Weltmer a modest $750 (Weltmer had sought $20,000), plus costs; the magazine got off altogether. Bishop appealed the decision to the Missouri Supreme Court, which at first seemed inclined to order a rehearing of the case. But in October 1902, the state's high court ruled that "a recent decision of the Supreme Court of the United States . . . announces a different conclusion as to the law from that declared in the case at bar."

In that case, Weltmer had sued J. M. McAnulty, Nevada's postmaster, who on orders from the postmaster general, acting on the complaints of physicians, had refused to deliver Weltmer's mail, returning letters stamped "fraudulent." The Supreme Court's ruling, finding Weltmer's practice in violation of no law of Congress and injoining the postmaster general from holding up Weltmer's mail, not only put a stop to the legal harassment but had the appearance of a blanket vindication of magnetic healing. In their opinions, some dissenting justices made sagacious comments about the mystery of mind-cure.

The lesser magnetic healers of Nevada ran the gamut. Some were undoubtedly quacks who laced their sessions with table-rappings, levitations, and mediumistic messages from the beyond; others deserved to be taken more seriously. Grant Harpold taught both barbering and magnetic healing in Harpold's Barbershop. The Marmaduke Institute, located at 128 South Main (actually a boardinghouse), bore a famed local and state name. In the East End, Professor and Mrs. A. A. Waddell held forth (he better known to Nevadans for his livery stable and she for her cancer-eaten nose, kept covered with a homemade cardboard nose); the neighborhood also hosted the Vito-Magnetic Sanitarium and the Hindoo School. Uptown, Professor J. C. Thurman and Mrs. S. R. Magnien (of the Eureka School) advertised "consulations free" in the *Nevada Daily Mail.* Professor T. B. Moss (of the Union School) boasted in the paper that he had been "alleviating pain for years" and was not only a hypnotist, a clairvoyant, and a horoscope writer but "connected with God."

Weltmer's toughest rival, however, was Leonard E. Stanhope (1860–19??), who brought an M.D. and a D.D.S. to his practice. Something of a one-man Nevada institution in his time, Stanhope was apparently not directly influenced by Weltmer. After a hard youth working on the railroad, by 1896 Stanhope had picked up his degrees (the M.D. from the Homeopathic Medical College of Missouri in St. Louis, in 1887) and was practicing medicine and surgery over his father's East End grocery store.

Old-timers recalled in a 1971 *Nevada Herald* report that a cloud always seemed to hang over Stanhope. Perhaps he failed to prosper at conventional medicine, although an entry, probably self-written, in *Encyclopedia of the History of Missouri,* says he was diverted by his sudden discovery of his own vast "magnetic" powers in the late 1890s. Whatever the circumstance, he became an instant expert on magnetic healing. His book *The Science of Magnetic Healing*—called "the standard work on the subject"—was published at Salina, Kansas, in 1898.

Coincidentally, in 1897, the very year Weltmer arrived, the Stanhope Sanitarium and School of Magnetic Healing opened in Nevada at 507 East Cherry—just across from Vito-Magnetic—in the limestone-quoin-trimmed brick mansion built by the late hardware tycoon J. A. Tyler.

Huge advertisements such as the following from the *Nevada Daily Mail* lauded the famous work and miracle cures of Stanhope and described his institution: "The spacious grounds cover one entire block on Nevada's most prominent street, yet well retired from the bustle of the city." "The building itself is a large, roomy brick, with wide porches on three sides of it, which are provided with easy rocking chairs for the patients. In the building are twelve large and conveniently arranged rooms, elegantly furnished and supplied with all modern conveniences." "The building is heated by steam and modern baths are at the command of the patients, the purest artesian water being used in the baths. For drinking water the Sanitarium is provided with the finest filtered cistern water."

The precise inner workings of the Weltmer Institute, the Stanhope Sanitarium, and other Nevada institutions based on magnetic healing are not well known. To many they were shrouded in an aura of alchemy and black magic. In the 1900 trial Bishop spoke of a man who died at the Stanhope Sanitarium whose body was smuggled out and onto a train at dawn. "My God, get that body out of here!" Stanhope was supposed to have implored the undertakers, who failed to confirm the tale. Of course, given the fact that many of the individuals who came to the magnetic healers may have been terminally ill and considered magnetic healing a last resort (Weltmer said 85 percent of his patients had been considered hopeless cases by doctors), it is plausible that patients could have died on the premises without cause being attributed to such institutions.

Most information about activities and treatments that took place at the magnetic healing institutions comes from the writings of the directors. Although Stanhope's book gives us more precise information about actual treatment procedures than Weltmer's more numerous and diffuse works, all the writings provide valuable insights into this fascinating field of healing. Photos of Stanhope in his books show a stocky, stolid-faced, small but imposing man with a leonine mustache, wearing a splendid frock coat and wing collar, dressed to command a patient's confidence—an important strategy for a healer, especially one using hypnotism. Weltmer had a similar presence.

"Magnetic healing," Stanhope wrote, "is classified into three subjects: hypnotism, vital magnetism, and mental science." And hypnotism, he remarked, "is the basic principle."

This statement was undoubtedly accurate for it is acknowledged that hypnotism, recognized as a medical tool since its discovery by Mesmer, is simply enhanced suggestibility, and suggestion proved to be the most valid and durable element of the Nevada movement. Interestingly, James Braid, a follower of Mesmer, inspired Charcot, the direct precursor of Freud, father of psychoanalysis. Long before Émile Coué gained fame in France by having his patients repeat "Day by day in every way I am feeling better and better," Weltmer shrewdly changed part of his institute's name from "Magnetic Healing" to "Suggestive Therapeutics."

Vital, or animal, magnetism, the second most important element employed by the institutions came, of course, directly from Mesmer. Both Weltmer and Stanhope—like Mesmer—held that all men have the power to heal by means of their "magnetism," or "life force"; that the miracle cures of religious leaders were simply examples of magnetic cures; and that the halos portrayed around their heads represented magnetic emanations. However, what Mesmer referred to as "fluidum," Weltmer called "man-effluvium" (hand outflow), although they meant basically the same phenomenon. In his magisterial 1913 work *The Practice of Suggestive Therapeutics* (Weltmerism's leatherbound, gold-leaf-edged, six-hundred-and-fifty-page "bible" presented to institute graduates), Ernest Weltmer readily acknowledged that "maneffluvium" and even "animal magnetism" were hypothetical, but he insisted that mind could still cure, via suggestion, whether such a physical basis existed or not.

Yet at the turn of the century, "magnetism" or "maneffluvium" were heavily relied on. Treatments resembled massages, or the religious "laying on of hands." *The Healing Hand,* a key Weltmer text, presented the idea that "touching is healing"—a phrase that, ironically, is the title of a 1982 mainstream medical work. And "magnetism" could be imparted in striking ways. "Magnetized" water might be prescribed for internal ailments; and a "magnetized" handkerchief could be mailed to a patient for application to an ailment.

Touching or other physical contact, however, were not of the essence. Treatment could be made through walls, or at a distance. For animal magnetism, even if not actually identical with thought, possessed thoughtlike properties—and can't thought travel anywhere instantly? In Weltmer's controversial "absent treatment," the patient simply made himself receptive at a prescribed hour, usually at rising or retiring, while the healer—who might be thousands of miles away—beamed out appropriate thought-waves.

Stanhope described the more down-to-earth "hands-on" treatment. First, he wrote, hang the hands downward to heat them by the rush of blood, then "make passes" over the seat of the trouble. To cure a headache, place the "positive" (right) hand on the forehead and the "negative" (left) one on the back and "send the current through." Then make passes over the head and down off the shoulders, giving "a quick little flip, exercising at the same time a strong intention to draw the pain out. If you do not take it off at the shoulders, you may get it down into the body and leave it there." Although Stanhope's description of giving treatment sounds fairly rudimentary, at the same time he warns prospective magnetic healers to have no illusions—it was harder work than it sounded. The healer was apt to wind up sweat-drenched and exhausted.

The third element used at the institutions was mental science, simply a fashionable name for faith. "The moment we realize our oneness with the Infinite Spirit, that moment we recognize that we are the masters of our bodies," said Stanhope. At a later time this would be described in such ways as "the power of positive thinking."

"Man has two distinct minds," Stanhope declared. "I prefer to call them the conscious and sub-conscious minds." It was this innate power in man that did the healing, Weltmer insisted; the healer merely sought to set it free. "It is the unconscious mind that must be aroused in all healings," he wrote in *The Healing Hand,* "for it is upon its actions that all healing depends.... The unconscious mind, or the healing mind— God's healing power in man—is the only healer of the ills of man. It is that force which has been called 'Nature' by physicians since the time of Hippocrates." It may increase our respect for the magnetic healers to recognize that this idea—so integral to the whole local movement—was put into print by a Nevadan a year before Sigmund Freud published the work that won him worldwide credit for it. At the time, the concept of the subconscious, or unconscious, mind was in the air.

For the first few years of their existence, the institutions flourished. Patients flocked to Nevada's healers, especially Weltmer. It looked as though Nevada would be the Lourdes of the future. However, since fashions in healing are almost as fickle as those of dress, the popularity of magnetic healing declined as rapidly as it had begun. Already by 1903 the roster of magnetic healers in the city directory had diminished to only three.

Weltmer, however, continued to prosper by changing with the times— altering the name of his institute to emphasize suggestive therapeutics rather than magnetic healing. Perhaps Stanhope was less flexible; at any rate, his heyday was brief, and he returned to conventional medicine. Although Stanhope's reputation had never been spotless, it apparently

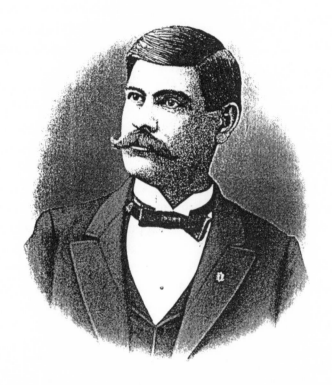

Dr. Leonard E. Stanhope, a graduate of the Homeopathic Medical College of Missouri, discovered his own "magnetic" powers in the late 1890s. Courtesy Bushwhacker Museum, Nevada, Missouri.

declined further after his sanitarium became less popular. For one thing his claim to be able to cure drug addiction was undermined by his own well-known uncured habit. Additionally, the location of his sanitarium was in the town's "tenderloin" district, where a doctor was expected to purvey certain timeless kinds of backstreet medical service. After Stanhope's death, his wife Eliza reportedly continued the service from the couple's home. To be seen coming out of Mrs. Stanhope's was the end of a girl's reputation.

Even though Weltmer was a very different sort of man, the controversy of 1900 concerning his institute has continued to simmer in Nevada. This can, in some measure, perhaps be attributed to jealousy on the part of less successful local physicians; in their 1900 brochure, the ministers had likened the magnetic healers to Demetrius of Ephesus, who made idols for the local shrine to Diana and was highly indignant when the Christian preachings of Paul put his livelihood in jeopardy. However, the Weltmer-anti-Weltmer controversy seems to have been grounded mainly in differing human temperaments: between those who hold that the human mind itself accurately reflects reality and those who believe the human mind is prone to self-deception and must be ruthlessly reined-in in favor of evidence gleaned by the senses and stern logic.

A comparison might be made with the famous Victorian quarrel between Cardinal Newman and "muscular Christian" Charles Kingsley over religious opinions. Each utterly, convincingly demolished the other's position in print. But, as to which individual won the debate, a commentator concludes it all depends on the kind of person you are. The hardheaded person who only believes in what can be seen will prefer Kingsley; while one who thinks human reason and the senses can be unreliable, that allowance must be made for mental or spiritual factors, will favor Newman. And so it was with the debate between Weltmer and the anti-Weltmerists. During their time, the scientific, rational view of the world was widely respected, but new developments were focusing on nonrational factors that could not be explained by contemporary scientific models. This was the era when Einstein, for instance, was about to explode Newtonian physics.

In the health field, physicians had long conceded that not all diseases are physically based, that some are merely "functional"—that is, symptoms exist where no organic disorder can be detected and are caused by a patient's mind. Mesmer himself had found it possible to make some symptoms disappear during hypnosis. And in our own day of emphasis on psychology, the skeptic's complaint that the magnetic healer's cures are "all in the mind" becomes ironic—as does Bishop's comparison of Weltmerism and "Negro voodoo and Christian Science." It is now generally recognized that Christian Science and even voodoo are systems wherein belief itself can produce physical effects not otherwise explainable.

Mrs. Roy C. Cunningham, a gentler critic of Weltmer, concedes that he was "an excellent hypnotist." "Some ailments he apparently treated successfully. The patients seemed fully recovered." He would hypnotize invalids, command them to walk, and they would do so—though such cures were not always permanent (a familiar feature of faith healing). These are examples of "functional," nonphysical illnesses caused by mental conditions which could successfully be treated by hypnosis. Much ridiculed by critics was Weltmer's and Stanhope's term "mental science"— meaning simply faith, faith in oneself or a higher spiritual being. From a modern perspective, it is evident that self-confidence heals.

"Weltmer recognized the need for medical care," writes Robert L. Stone, Jr. "He advocated the use of surgery if a person needed it. He never assumed that he could cure everyone. He never claimed to have miraculous powers."

This modesty and larger perspective is probably what helped Weltmer prosper and survive. A movement such as magnetic healing could easily attract charlatans who indeed would abuse it and claim to cure everyone. It is revealing that Weltmer's imitators faded from the scene quickly, while he went on doing business at the same institute until his death of old age in 1930. By then, he had advised three million individuals by mail and issued some half a million diplomas. His institute annually hosted the conventions of the American Association of Suggestive Therapeutics, and he addressed state associations around the country. His son Ernest, though unable to keep the institute going through the Depression, continued to write and lecture on psychotherapy until his own death in the 1950s. Although a local legend persists that Weltmer was under indictment for mail fraud at the time of his death and that the institute shut down for that reason, this is not true. The mail fraud case— a sixteen-day "stop order" on his mail which was lifted after personal exoneration from the postmaster general—occurred twenty-eight years prior to Weltmer's death. Clearly the institute closed simply on account of its guiding spirit's death, coupled with changes in the times and in the fickle fashions of medical care.

Not widely known is the fact that Weltmer's interests went beyond therapeutics. Although no reference can be found to the "Weltmer Experiment" of 1907–1910 under the concept of "telepathy" in an encyclopedia, Weltmer conducted "perhaps the best-known series of experiments in telepathy conducted by investigators in America," according to William Walker Atkinson in his 1910 book *Telepathy: Its Theory, Facts, and Proof.* At the time, Weltmer was vice president of a New Thought group and regularly interacted with the New Thought movement, which published Atkinson's book. It contains three chapters on the Weltmer Experiment and praises Sidney and Ernest Weltmer for their "frankness and fairness" in their effort to prove or disprove telepathy. The landmark Duke Experiments of 1930 merely duplicated Weltmer's fascinating if inconclusive results.

From our present-day perspective, Weltmer seems to have been just what Robert L. Stone, Jr., called him in his dissertation, a "pioneer of psychotherapy," of thoroughly honest motives. It was a day when orthodox medicine was reacting to innovation and daring, even in its own ranks, with witch-hunting savagery. In many ways, Weltmer was simply ahead of his time. As Dr. William S. Brink, executive director of the American Association of Professional Hypnotherapists, wrote in 1984, "What was being written seventy-five years ago is for the most part what is being written today. Today it just gets dressed up in high-tech jargon, which makes it sound something altogether new."

While the term "magnetic healing" is likely permanently out of favor, the ideas of Mesmer—as of Weltmer and Stanhope—are still very much alive. In the late 1940s, Freudian psychologist Wilhelm Reich rehabilitated the idea of "fluidum" under a new name: "orgone." Dozens of thinkers still defend the reality of some mesmeric "life force." And in recent years there has been a revival of the old Chinese therapy of acupuncture, based on the theory of "yin" and "yang"—in many respects uncannily like the "positive" and "negative" of the magnetic healers.

To quote the oft-ridiculed motto of Mesmer himself, "Much will rise again that has long been buried."

BIBLIOGRAPHIC ESSAY

The author is curator at the Bushwhacker Museum in Nevada, Missouri, where much of the source material for this essay is housed, including unpublished manuscripts such as "Weltmer: Pioneer of Psychotherapy" by Robert Lowell Stone, Jr. (undated dissertation, no academic provenience); "The History of the Development of Medical Care in Vernon County from 1844 to 1987" by Warren C. Lovinger, M.D. (1987); an untitled, undated manuscript by Mrs. Roy C. Cunningham; a 1994 letter to the author from Clay Bailey, St. Andrews, Tennessee, quoting *Nautilus* 44 (November 1916); and a 1984 letter to the author from William S. Brink, Ph.D.

Museum archives contain many illuminating vintage publications on magnetic healing, such as the following: *The Healing Hand* by Sidney A. Weltmer (Nevada, Mo.: Weltmer Foundation, 1925); *How to Make Magnetic Healing Pay* by Sidney A. Weltmer (Kansas City, Mo.: Hudson-Kimberly Publishing Co., 1901); *The Science of Magnetic Healing* by Leonard E. Stanhope, M.D., D.D.S. (Salina, Kan.: Central Kansas Publishing Co., 1899); *The Magnetic Healer's Guide* by J. O. Crone (Kansas City, Mo.: Hudson-Kimberly Publishing Co., 1903); *The Practice of Suggestive Therapeutics* by Ernest Weltmer (Nevada, Mo.: Weltmer Institute of Suggestive Therapeutics, 1913); "Empiricism in Missouri and How to Suppress It" by E. L. Priest, M.D., *The Kansas City Medical Index-Lancet* (July 1899); and issues of the *Magnetic Journal* (Nevada, Mo.: American School of Magnetic Healing).

Other local history materials include *Wassum's City Directory of Nevada, Missouri* (Nevada, Mo.: Lang and Young, 1900 and 1903 editions) and *Encyclopedia of the History of Missouri* (New York, N.Y., Louisville, Ky., and St. Louis, Mo.: Southern Historical Co., 1901). The author consulted the following legal archives: "In the Supreme Court of Missouri, Div. #1, April Term, 1902; S. A. Weltmer and J. H. Kelly, Respondents, vs. C. M. Bishop, Appellant; Appealed from Bates County Circuit Court"; Ditto: "Appellent's Statement, Points, and Argument; M. T. January, of Counsel for Appellant"; Ditto: "Respondent's Statements, Points and Argument; Francisco and Clark, Scott and Bowker, Attorneys for Respondents." The following legal record was also utilized: U. S. Supreme Court: *American School of Magnetic Healing v. J. M.*

McAnulty. *United States Reports* 187; *Lawyer's Edition* 47; *Supreme Court Reporter* 23.

Other works consulted include *Franz Anton Mesmer: Between God and Devil* by James Wyckoff (New York: Prentice Hall, 1975); *Mesmerism and the American Cure of Souls* by Robert C. Fuller (Philadelphia: University of Pennsylvania Press, 1982); *Spiritism* by E. H. Estabrooks (New York: Dutton, 1947); *Ancient Wisdom Revealed* by Bruce F. Campbell (Berkeley: University of California Press, 1980); *The Inland Ground: An Evocation of the American Middle West* by Richard Rhodes (New York: Atheneum, 1970); *The Practice of Autosuggestion by the Method of Émile Coué* by C. Harry Brooks (London: Allen & Unwin, 1922); *The Positive Thinkers* by Donald Meyer (Middletown, Conn.: Wesleyan University Press, 1988); *Touching Is Healing* by Jules Older (New York: Stein & Day, 1982); *The Interpretation of Dreams* by Sigmund Freud, translated by James Strachey (New York: Avon Books, 1965); *Devils, Drugs, and Doctors* by Howard W. Haggard, M.D. (New York: Harper, 1929); *Telepathy: Its Theory, Facts, and Proof* by William Walker Atkinson (Chicago: New Thought Publishing Company, 1910); *Extra-Sensory Perception* by J. B. Rhine (Boston: Bruce Humphries, 1935); and *Fury on Earth: A Biography of Wilhelm Reich* by Myron Sharaf (New York: St. Martin's Press, 1983).

Photocopied and bound facsimile editions of some of the magnetic healing texts produced by the Weltmers and other Nevada practitioners are available from Health Research, Box 70, Mokelumne Hill, CA 95245.

The Milling Brothers: Texas "Outlaw" Medicine Men

GENE FOWLER

"THE DAY OF MYSTERY" proclaimed the headline of an advertisement in the *Cisco* (Texas) *Apert* of July 27, 1905. "Dr. R. G. Milling, the renowned Magnetic healer or drugless doctor, is now in Cisco. His power over disease is well known all over the state...."

"MYSTERY OF MYSTERIES" headlined an ad in the *Cisco Round-up*. "All chronic diseases yield to the power of Dr. Milling. From whence comes this mysterious power or how it is derived is not known."

Sometimes billed as "The Indian Adept" or "The Long-Haired Doctor," Roscoe Gorman Milling (1868–1925) had arrived in Texas from his native Georgia around 1890, settling first in Stephenville, southwest of Fort Worth. Younger brother George (G. R.) Milling (1874–1914) followed later. Shunning the barber's chair, the brothers presented a Wild West image to early twentieth-century Texans, calling on their part-Cherokee heritage to boost their mystique as medicine men.

Like many who sought to build up America's turn-of-the-century "vitality," R. G. Milling had familiarized himself with the tenets of Weltmerism, but the "Milling Method" he developed (and taught younger brother G. R. and many others) seems to have been his own combination of massage, faith healing, hypnotism, and showmanship.

Tales passed to Milling's descendants, many of whom became chiropractors, naturopaths, and M.D.s, relate that he first experienced the gift of healing as a small boy in Georgia. His mother suffered from phlebitis, and the best physicians of Atlanta could not provide relief. Desperate to comfort her, young Milling began to rub the woman, as though driven by a sense that he could draw the sickness out of her body. To everyone's astonishment, she recovered quickly.

The family acquired a medical library for the bright, surprising child, and he began to learn about the maladies to which flesh is heir. Like many other American boys in the 1880s, however, as a teenager Milling felt the urge to wander out west. Family lore contends that he ran off with Buffalo Bill's Wild West troupe, traveling with the show for an indefinite period of time. If the story is true, the magnetic Milling doubtless picked up valuable tips on showmanship from the buckskinned impresario.

After he settled in Stephenville in 1890, the "rubbing doctor" sidelined in his second favorite preoccupation, agriculture. Descendants recall family stories of his experiments with terracing for soil conservation, reportedly the earliest such efforts in Erath County.

At some point a visit to nearby Glen Rose augumented his continuing medical education when the Indian Adept witnessed a Hindu hypnotist demonstrating his esoteric technique for a circle of local youths. "Dressed in the toga traditional with Oriental mystics," reported the *Wichita Falls Record News*, the Hindu hypnotist passed his hands over the Glen Rose youths' faces, uttered the "hypnotic jargon that's reputed to turn the trick, and while the hypnotized clients mumbled and slept, young Milling's eyes almost popped from their sockets simultaneous with the birth of a creative impulse to do something for humanity."

After his first wife Ella died during childbirth in 1904, Milling moved on to practice for a time in Rising Star, before "The Day of Mystery" arrived in Cisco. East of Abilene, Cisco would later gain fame as the site of Conrad Hilton's first hotel and for a bank robbery pulled just before Christmas by a man dressed as Santa Claus.

In another *Cisco Round-up* ad, the Indian Adept compared his treatment to the self-medication of man's best friend: "When a dog gets sick he eats a little grass and gets well. When man gets sick he absorbs a concoction of drastic drugs and ruins his stomach. The dog sticks to the treatment which nature has provided—simple and harmless, but effective. Dr. Milling heals without medicine, the natural way."

"His treatment is the only safe and reliable treatment," proclaimed another ad, "which acts at once upon the nerve forces, stopping the drain and replacing the wornout and run-down tissues; it increases the weight in sound healthy flesh and muscles that give strength, and fills the brain

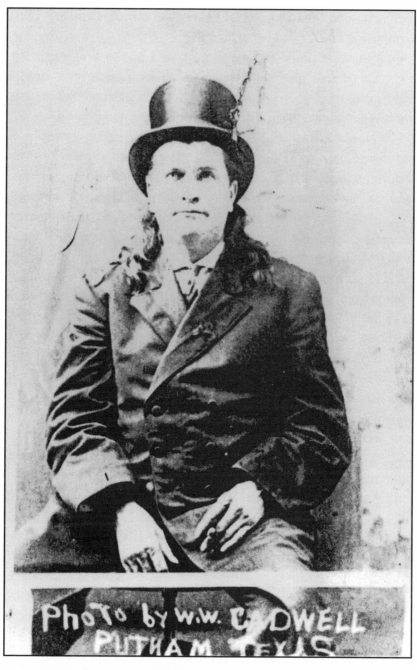

Photo by W.W. CALDWELL
PUTNAM TEXAS

Magnetic healer R. G. Milling, known as the Long-Haired Doctor and
the Indian Adept, administered drugless treatments to thousands
of Texans from 1890 to 1925.
Photo circa 1912, courtesy Ova Withee, Irving, Texas, and Ida Mae Waddell,
Putnam, Texas.

with nerve and fresh vitality building up the entire system and transforming the sufferer into perfect health."

According to family tradition, at least one Cisco resident sought the services of Milling in secret, not wanting fellow citizens to know that he had resorted to a "rubbing doctor." But after the man improved, he went door-to-door, spreading the magnetic manifesto through town.

By June of 1907, the Long-Haired Doctor's offices had moved from the City Hotel to the Eppler House. The *Cisco Round-up* carried a series of advertisements that sounded an alarm: "All the sick and lame of Eastland and adjoining counties, who have dosed themselves with nostrums without relief and who in vain have sacrificed their hopes upon the altar of homeopathy, should see at once Dr. Milling, the famous drugless healer, before it is everlastingly too late."

The cause of such urgency was a tightening of Texas's medical licensing regulations, set to take effect on July 12. "The gift of magnetic healing was dispensing the boon of health to thousands whom medicine could not reach," the ad continued, "and a new era was dawning for ailing humanity, when this law stepped in and said that the old method of saw and knife and pill-bags was good enough." After July 12, the ads solemnly proclaimed, Milling would quit practice. "If you ever expect to get well, if you do not want the pill-bag route for a long journey into an unknown land, you will have to hurry.... Dr. Milling has been in Cisco two years, and in this county he has built a monument to his memory that will live forever.... In this land of the setting sun thousands of hearts are attuned with the throbbing stress of life renewed to sing his praise."

After the new law took effect, Milling moved his second wife Lenora and their seven children to the country north of Cisco (possibly near Eliasville) and returned to farming. As descendants relate, however, folks tracked the popular healer down and camped in wagons on the farm. They pleaded for treatment, and Milling could not turn them away. The Indian Adept became an outlaw medicine man.

Milling's trail picks up next in the fall of 1910 near the small community of Gunsight, named for the Gunsight Mountains north of Cisco. His notices in the *Eastland Chronicle* offered "good beds and plenty of cover, with pork chops greasy" at his new hotel in Gunsight. Room and board was $2 a day, but scientific masseur treatment was free.

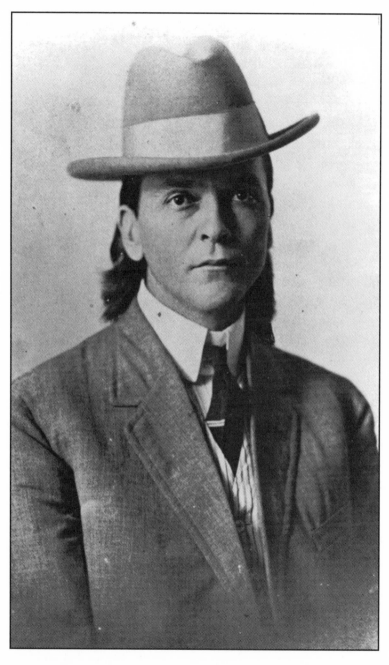

R. G. Milling's younger brother, G. R. Milling, practiced magnetic healing in Glen Rose, Texas, from 1911 to 1914, when he was killed on the town square, possibly by the angry husband of a female patient.
Photo courtesy Texas Christian University Press.

One who visited the country sanitarium that November was R. L. McFall of Breckenridge. The following July, in 1911, McFall took the stand in the Stephens County courthouse in Breckenridge to testify that Milling had practiced medicine on him without a license. Describing Milling's treatment for rheumatism, McFall stated, as quoted in the transcript of the case's appeal: "He placed his right hand on my nose and his left hand at the back of my head and then he rubbed his hands up and down my body and to below my knees and clasped his hands around my knee that was affected. When I stood up, I found that the soreness and pain in my knee was almost gone."

His rheumatism at least temporarily relieved, McFall seems to have been more upset by the $2 meal price at Milling's than with the fact that the Indian Adept was not a licensed physician. "I ate dinner with Dr. Milling," he testified. "I am acquainted with the kind, grade, quantity, and quality of meals that is ordinarily served in this country at hotels and boarding houses and for which 25 cents is charged. It was an ordinary 25 cent meal. I did not leave my home and go to Dr. Milling's for the purpose of eating dinner with him. I went there for treatment."

When Milling took the stand, he confirmed that he had treated McFall but only "within [his] particular sphere of labor as a Masseur." The $2 charge was for board and lodging, including stables for guests' teams, which Milling judged to be "well worth $2 a day." Nevertheless, the jury found the outlaw healer guilty, fined him $50, and sentenced him to twenty minutes in jail.

But even the loss of the case's appeal in 1912 failed to deter Milling; it may in fact have spurred him to become more vocal in promoting his practice. By the time the appeal was denied in Austin, the renegade practitioner had relocated to Putnam, between Cisco and Abilene on the Texas & Pacific Railroad line. Handbills for Putnam's Hotel Milling Sanitarium identified him as "The Renowned Healer!" Noting that the West Texas resort was equipped with steam heat and electric lighting, the flyer promised "free masseur treatment" and "free mineral water" for a $3 per day hotel rate.

In a brochure published in March 1912, the Indian Adept described his healing philosophy by comparing the human body to a subirrigated farm: "A farmer finds his tank running over, but part of the farm is very dry, and part very wet." To correct this circulatory problem, the farmer calls in a medical doctor, who tells the farmer to pour a bushel of lime into the tank three times a day. Next, a surgeon cuts off one of the pumps. When the crops keep withering, the farmer consults a Christian Scientist. "Just forget you have a farm, and God will take care of it," advises the Christian Scientist. "As a man thinketh in his heart, so is he."

A "Suggestive Therapeutist" tries to correct the water flow with affirmations and positive thinking. The farmer "has been reading about Dr. Still's wonderful Institute, and now he calls an osteopath." He makes osteopathic adjustments on the irrigation line, but still the farm deteriorates. Then a chiropractor thumps on the main pipe three minutes a day for a week. Finally, the farmer finds a blind Japanese masseur.

"I have spent all my money, lost all my religion, and almost lost my farm," the farmer tells the blind masseur. "But if you will do something for my farm I will pay you if I ever get any money." The blind masseur follows the water's flow down the main pipe and along the internal pipes, removing obstructions where he finds the ground too dry, restoring full circulation to the irrigation system.

Editors, merchants, the justice of the peace, and other prominent Putnam citizens allowed their names to be published in the brochure as an endorsement of the Indian Adept, and two dozen testimonials by satisfied patients from Cisco and surrounding towns told of cures for rheumatism, neuralgia, appendicitis, gallstones, "the morphine habit," and other maladies. A lady from Morgan advised all sufferers to "throw away your medicine and go to Dr. Milling."

Gordon, Texas, resident John Boyd Harlin recalled the time Milling healed his older brother T. M. Harlin. "It was sometime before 1915," he remembered, "and my brother got too hot one day playing baseball. He got infantile paralysis. The doctors said he would never walk again, and my dad, you know, he was just grabbin' at straws, so he took my brother to see Dr. Milling in Putnam. Dr. Milling had him up and walking in three days." Harlin couldn't remember the exact nature of the treatment—Milling either massaged his brother's muscles or made "magnetic" passes over his body, or perhaps a combination of the two. His brother had a slight limp thereafter, said Harlin, but he lived

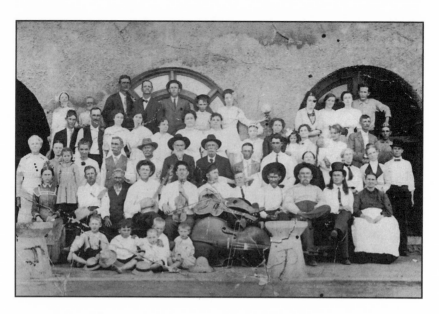

R. G. Milling, musicians, and patients at Hotel Milling Sanitarium,
Putnam, Texas, circa 1912.
Photo courtesy Ova Withee, Irving, Texas.

to the age of seventy-two, putting in full days of work at the family grocery store. The family kept the "Renowned Healer's" flyer for seventy-five years.

Apparently, opposition followed Milling wherever he went. Dr. Solon Milton of Putnam sent a copy of the brochure to the Bureau of Investigation at the American Medical Association in Chicago. "It would be impossible," replied the AMA's Dr. Arthur J. Cramp in a letter to Milton, "for a man of Milling's physiognomy to be anything but a quack. He evidently belongs to that gradually disappearing, long-haired type that used to be so common."

Callahan County historian John Berry provided a more sympathetic portrait of the magnetic healer's presence in Putnam. "Dr. Milling was a picturesque character and willing to put forth effort and time to add to the picturesqueness and to remain a character," wrote Berry in the 1963 *West Texas Historical Association Yearbook.* "He was a handsome man with a distinguished air about him. He wore a frock-tailed coat and his long hair reached to his shoulders. He was a convincing talker and a striking figure."

The Indian Adept's Putnam sanitarium was housed in a sixty-room, Spanish Mission-style hotel opened in 1910 as the Carter-Holland. When Milling sold it around 1917, it became known as the Mission Hotel. As historian Berry reminisced, a stay at the stuccoed sanitarium could be very pleasant: "An orchestra was kept to furnish background music for all occasions and to help soothe the nerves of the many patients who came to drink the water and take the baths and treatments. Various groups negotiated with them to play for dances, usually held on Saturday night or on special occasions. The ball room floor was of maple. It was beautiful and also very slick when a little corn meal was added." Granddaughter Ova Withee recalled that the dances often featured fiddle bands from nearby Ranger. Patients posed for postcard photos outside the sanitarium with the Long-Haired Doctor and musicians.

By 1917, R. G. Milling was based back in Cisco. *The Way to Health without Drugs or the Knife,* a twenty-four-page booklet printed on *Cisco Round-up* presses that year, provided further explanation of magnetism and testimonial defense to the "severe and well-organized opposition" to his practice.

Magnetism, wrote the rebel masseur, "is a power or force so subtle and yet so potential that to measure its breadth and depth, and to ascertain all its uses and purposes, would require more years than are allotted to man on this earth, for its possibilities are unlimited." He described the application and development of this "infinite energy from which all things proceed" in terms of early twentieth-century advances in transportation, communication, and standard of living. And he compared the "operating table with the horrid nightmare of the ether or chloroform" to past centuries when "snake bones, toads' blood, human hair and human flesh were used as great remedies."

Refuting "all efforts to decry, belittle or ridicule [himself] or [his] system," *The Way to Health without Drugs or the Knife* stated that eight thousand "chronic cases" had been treated by the system, and that "only six people have been carried out of [his] Sanitariums dead, and [Milling's] friends know their condition when they came."

The drugless doctor relocated a final time around 1920, when he moved about sixty miles east to the health resort city of Mineral Wells, widely known as the home of Crazy Water, a native elixir that allegedly cured a pioneer woman of insanity. There, R. G. Milling assisted at the sanitarium of eldest son H. H. Milling, one of many descendants and in-laws trained in the Milling Method by the Indian Adept.

The part-Cherokee magnetic healer must have softened his rigid views of mainstream surgical medicine toward the end of his life. When a kidney ailment stumped his powers in 1925, he checked into Dallas's Baylor Hospital, where he died in April from complications following an operation.

Younger brother G. R. Milling met an even less pleasant end eleven years earlier in Glen Rose, where he established a sanitarium in 1911. The town must have seemed a magical place when he first arrived. Nestled near the Paluxy River amid gently-sloping limestone hills, the oak-, cedar-, and cottonwood-shaded jewel of a village presented a geologic wonderland. Well-preserved dinosaur tracks, discovered just a few years earlier, lay in the bed of the Paluxy and the nearby countryside. Stands of petrified wood added to the atmosphere, as well as hundreds of bubbling springs and artesian wells. On many spring and summer evenings, music and laughter wafted across the Paluxy from a lighted party barge called the Floating Palace. A crumbling cabin on the edge of town recalled John

St. Helen, a mysterious resident of the early 1870s rumored to have actually been John Wilkes Booth.

Tonkawas and other Indians had long used the area as a place of healing, restoring themselves with the purgative sulphur water. By the 1870s, settlers had discovered the natural tonic, and in fair weather the little valley was dotted with covered wagons camped for the waters. Patrons of the Sans Souci Bar could balance their firewater intake with liberal gulps of healthful white sulphur water, as a "perpetually-flowing Artesian fountain" in the saloon dispensed the local elixir free of charge.

Though Glen Rose never acquired a rail connection, the water and the area's natural beauty made it a popular health and pleasure resort with many parks and sanitariums. G. R. Milling had probably read the 1900 U.S. Geological Survey report judging the Glen Rose waters "valuable for medicinal purposes" and more like the waters of Carlsbad, Austria, "than any other mineral water." A Glen Rose brochure of the era was more modest, calling the restorative beverage "not a curative water in the ordinary accepted sense, but a remarkable system-builder, found to be a blend of White Sulphur, Black Sulphur, Magnesia, Iron and Chalbete." Whatever its efficacy, local bootleggers found the water made dandy moonshine after the town voted dry around 1902.

At first, G. R. Milling's practice flourished in Glen Rose. Soon after his arrival, he established a sanitarium on a block of land near the Methodist Church. A typical advertisement from a 1912 issue of the *Glen Rose Reporter* boasts of the marvelous improvement of a Sweetwater woman after two weeks at the Milling Sanitarium. The lady had been ill for four years, and "the best physicians had given her case up as a hopeless one." Other ads in the same issue touted the glories of somewhat more traditional panaceas like Simmons' Liver Purifier, Hunt's Lightning Oil, and Texas Wonder. Manufactured in St. Louis, Texas Wonder promised to cure diabetes and remove gravel from the bladder.

Somervell County courthouse files reveal that the sheriff was a frequent visitor to the sanitarium—but not for treatment. Charges lodged against G. R. Milling ranged from driving his Hupmobile down Barnard Street in excess of the 18 mph speed limit to disturbing a religious congregation. Five times he was charged with the unlicensed practice of medicine. Glen Rose attorney Levi Herring eased him out of those charges by arguing that masseurs were exempt from medical licensing statutes and that Milling practiced a massage treatment only. On five other occasions the magnetic healer was nabbed for toting a pistol in town and once for "unlawfully shooting a gun across a public road." In yet another charge the doctor allegedly threatened to take a life. A few cases involved his going on a bender.

County authorities agreed to a package deal in June 1914, dismissing several cases and accepting a guilty plea for several others. But conflict between the placid community and the independent-spirited healer continued. The tension boiled over in the lingering heat of late summer, just a few days after Milling's latest charge for practicing medicine without a license. At 11:30 A.M. on Wednesday, September 9, 1914, W. T. Newman, a farmer from the small community of Fairy (about thirty miles south), shot and killed the forty-year-old healer near the courthouse with blasts from a double-barreled shotgun.

A report on the shooting in the *Stephenville Empire* stated that Newman "gave himself over to the sheriff as the man that did the shooting." Perhaps indicative of G. R. Milling's stormy relationship with fellow townsmen, Newman's $3,500 bond was "furnished in a few minutes by several Glen Rose parties." The *Empire* story said a grand jury would weigh the evidence in November, but the case file is missing from courthouse archives, and no press coverage has been located with the final disposition of the case.

Newman's testimony in the examining trial indicated that the shooting stemmed from "family trouble." Contemporary Glen Rose historians only know that it had something to do with a woman. Remembering that magnetic healers were sometimes called "rubbing doctors" might suggest a number of scenarios.

Older brother R. G. Milling's youngest son, R. G. Milling, Jr., offered the Milling Method at a Glen Rose sanitarium well into the 1960s, closing down about the same time that Eastland County historian Pearl Ghormley was interviewing old-timers in Cisco. They remembered R. G. Milling, Sr., as "quite a curiosity," walking the streets of Cisco with his long, flowing hair and black silk top hat and Indian headband.

Some told stories of the outlaw healer's magical powers, a claim repeated in a Ripley's Believe-It-Or-Not feature nearly half a century after the drugless doctor's merger with "the changes called death." Along with drawings and text describing "The ALTAR OF BOU NOUARA in Algeria, which appears to be the statue of a supine human…built by cavemen 20,000 years ago" and "The LEFT HANDED WHELK, a shell…used by American Indians as a ceremonial cup," that day's feature included the following amazing-but-true item with accompanying illustration: "DR. ROSCOE GORMAN MILLING of Cisco, Texas, who taught himself hypnotism in the 19th Century, WOULD TOUCH A GLASS OF WATER AND CONVINCE A PATIENT IT WAS AN EFFECTIVE MEDICINE."

BIBLIOGRAPHIC ESSAY

Much information was obtained from interviews with R. G. Milling's granddaughter, naturopath Ova Withee of Irving, Texas; R. G. Milling's grandson, chiropractor H. Chief Brown of Cisco, Texas; and R. G. Milling, Jr.'s, widow, Alta McWilliams of Cleburne, Texas. Ova Withee provided photos, *The Way to Health without Drugs or the Knife,* and other miscellaneous documents. Thanks also to Mary Jo Deen Vague of Houston and Revvie Lee Hefner Neaves of Spur, Texas. Larry L. King reminisces briefly about R. G. Milling in "Requiem for a West Texas Town," in *Warning: Writer at Work* (Fort Worth: Texas Christian University Press, 1985). Pearl Ghormley's notes on R. G. Milling appear in *Eastland County, Texas: A Historical and Biographical Survey* (Austin, Tex.: Rupegy Publishing Co., 1969). G. R. Milling appears briefly in *Somervell, Story of a Texas County* by W. C. Nunn (Fort Worth: Texas Christian University Press, 1975). R. G. Milling's obituary, on file at the Boyce Ditto Library in Mineral Wells, Texas, also proved useful.

I interviewed John Boyd Harlin in Gordon, Texas, in 1990, and he presented me with the Milling flyer his family had kept for seventy-five years. The Hotel Milling Sanitarium brochure from Putnam, Texas, 1912, is on file in the Alternative Medicine and Health Fraud Collection at the American Medical Association, Chicago, along with letters inquiring about Milling descendants into the 1950s. A number of photographs of R. G. Milling are exhibited at the Conrad Hilton Memorial Park and Community Center museum (housed in Conrad Hilton's first hotel) in Cisco, Texas, and a photo of G. R. Milling is on view at Somervell County Museum in Glen Rose, Texas. Portions of this chapter appeared in *Crazy Water* by Gene Fowler (Fort Worth: Texas Christian University Press, 1991).

Buffalo Bill's Medicine Man: Dr. Frank "White Beaver" Powell

Eric V. Sorg

"One of the biggest liars God ever let live" was how a North Platte, Nebraska, newspaper described him in 1898, and Baron Münchausen and P. T. Barnum would have warmed to a kindred spirit. Nevertheless, when all was said and done, few dared challenge the wildly exaggerated claims of Frank Powell, the "Medicine Chief of the Winnebagos." No matter how free he might have been with the facts, he was still a brilliant doctor.

Like his future "blood brother," Buffalo Bill Cody, David Franklin Powell (1847–1906) became the male head of his household at the age of nine when his father, Dr. C. H. Powell, died; Isaac Cody died from complications of a wound that he received when Bill was nine. Young Powell immediately started working in a pharmacy in his hometown of Bethel, New York, which later led to pharmacy positions in Chicago, Illinois, and Omaha, Nebraska, where he received a beneficiary scholarship to the Louisville Medical College. Powell studied at the medical college for two years, graduated with honors on February 28, 1873, and within the next month accepted a position as a contract surgeon at Fort McPherson, Nebraska. Among his medical charges were the troops stationed at William "Buffalo Bill" Cody's hometown of North Platte, Nebraska. It was a happy stroke of luck for both men. Buffalo Bill, who had launched his acting career in Chicago just four months earlier, enjoyed coming home to relax in the congenial company of the young doctor. Both men shared a fondness for drink, cigars, hunting, telling stories, and adventure, and both were blessed with egos of respectable dimension.

After completing his Fort McPherson contract in 1877, Powell set up practice in Lanesboro, Minnesota. It was near there that he acquired the nickname White Beaver and began to style himself Medicine Chief of the Winnebagos. In the years to come, Powell spread information about

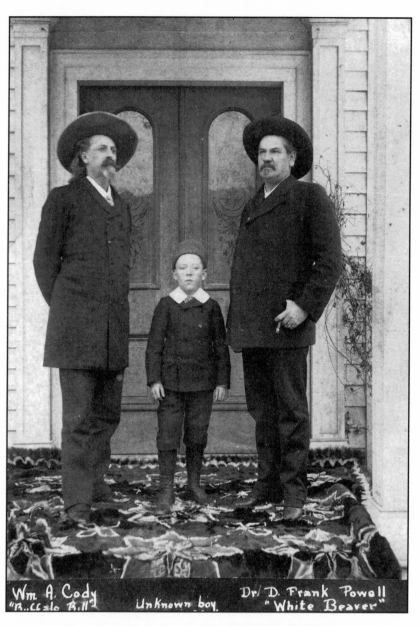

Wm. A. Cody "Buffalo Bill"   Unknown boy.   Dr. D. Frank Powell "White Beaver"

Dr. Frank Powell, known as White Beaver and the Medicine Chief of the
Winnebagos, with his friend and associate Buffalo Bill Cody
Photo courtesy Murphy Library, University of Wisconsin at La Crosse,
neg. no. 19497.

himself liberally over the regional print media, both in advertisements and in "articles" and "news stories" that he paid for. But neither he nor his brothers George and William, also doctors, left behind any papers, other than public records. Years later, Powell would exercise power of attorney for Buffalo Bill. However, while he is frequently mentioned as being in the Cody entourage, there are few references to Powell in Buffalo Bill's own extensive archives.

During the second week in August 1881, Buffalo Bill and his friend Powell went to the La Crosse, Wisconsin, area for an extended trip among the Winnebagos, auditioning Indians for Buffalo Bill's show of the season, *The Prairie Waif.* They signed two of the sons—Moses and Jake—of the Winnebago woman Four Deer Decorah, along with the "Indian Princess Wench-Tsha (Straight Talker)" and Charlie Medicine Smoke. Medicine Smoke's father was Winneshiek, head chief of the Winnebagos and one of the men credited with bestowing the name White Beaver on Powell. When Winneshiek died five months later, the *La Crosse Morning Chronicle* reported that Medicine Smoke would probably succeed his father unless several of the older chiefs stopped "the pretender to authority."

The cast of *The Prairie Waif* rehearsed in nearby Lanesboro, resulting in the folk belief that Buffalo Bill's Wild West started there, and opened in Davenport, Iowa, on September 1. The theatrical combination had some rough areas to work out—when they played in Chicago, Cody and Powell fought with the Winnebagos in the theater's green room—but they had solid bookings until the tour closed in May.

The Prairie Waif played well in La Crosse in spite of the conflicts, a reworking of earlier scripts, and as the *La Crosse Morning Chronicle* stated, a "slovenliness in speaking suggestive of a very mediocre stage manager." For the opening in La Crosse, press agent John M. ("Arizona John") Burke and White Beaver Powell concocted a story that while Deputy Grand Master Mason for Nebraska, Colorado, and Wyoming, Powell had made Cody a Master Mason. This hoopla, together with the publicity from the recruiting trip, effectively introduced White Beaver Powell to the La Crosse public, and within two months he moved his medical practice there.

Powell advertised his practice extensively. His costs were not only for traditional ads, which often stated "No Cure, No Pay," but also for "news stories" about himself, for which he paid 12 to 50 cents per line. In addition to his superb skills as a doctor, Powell catered to his clients' needs with house calls, a telephone line, and an all-night emergency service. By early 1882, Powell had doubled his office space and contacted his brothers George and William to join him.

Powell's career was punctuated with repeated attacks by rival practitioners on his credibility and numerous defenses of his abilities in the local press. White Beaver's treatment methods were questioned because, unlike most of the doctors of that era, Powell did not follow a single methodology. Moreover, he used herbs and Indian homeopathy, which opened his practice to professional scorn. Powell offered his detractors a challenge in the *La Crosse Morning Chronicle*, declaring: "I will take five of the worst cases of rupture…of any kind and will cure out of the above number of selected cases, four without danger to life and without the use of the knife or any other harsh or barbarous treatment, provided, first, that the patients follow my instructions, which will be neither impossible or hard to follow…. Second, each patient cured shall pay to me in money or its equivalent the sum of one hundred dollars." Powell offered to pay for his clients' time if he failed, but he wanted nothing from the doctors if he succeeded. Nobody picked up the gauntlet.

Over the next few months Powell's medical ads became subdued, and articles pertaining to his incredible skill with firearms appeared. Some of these undoubtedly were authored by Powell, but the *Morning Chronicle's* review of the Cole Brothers' Circus performance in July stated that most of the shooting routine of the Bogardus family (Captain A. H. Bogardus was called America's champion pigeon shot) could have been duplicated by Powell with a small-caliber pistol.

Powell knew the value of name recognition and continued to keep his name in the newspapers with reports of his operations and various activities. His friendship with Cody added to his glamour, and he acted as Buffalo Bill's self-appointed local spokesman. In this way, White Beaver was able to link his name with news items such as Cody's unsuccessful negotiations with Sitting Bull to tour with "Buffalo Bill's Combination" during the 1882 season. But all this publicity was not without its drawbacks. Certain people resented White Beaver and made threats against him.

Some support for Powell was shown by the *Morning Chronicle* on September 18: "The success of Doctor D. F. Powell, widely known as

White Beaver, has been phenomenal. Few members of the profession have stepped into a field of work, such as La Crosse, and acquired so immediately an uppermost round in the ladder of professional ability and uninterrupted prosperity…he is frank to a fault and discriminates in favor to no one, be he great and rich, or unknown and poor."

Many of the poor that Powell ministered to were the Winnebagos, who were treated free of charge by their "medicine chief." White Beaver's powerful influence over his Indian friends did not go unnoticed. In mid-October Powell successfully pacified the Winnebagos when they threatened to become violent during the trial of Charles Carter for the murder of Little George. As the result of his intervention, the *La Crosse Morning Chronicle* reported, "No trouble is now feared."

Around New Year's Day, articles once again ran in national and local papers about Powell's proficiency with firearms. *Cheek* magazine ran a long article on Powell's shooting ability in December 1882, stating that as a marksman Powell's skill was equal or superior to that of Cody, William Frank Carver, and A. H. Bogardus. And in January 1883, the *La Crosse News* ran another long article on Powell's ability titled "Bad Man with a Gun." Some believe Powell engineered the spate of articles on his firearms prowess to scare into silence people in the medical community who were slandering him. However, if this was the case, it did not work. The attacks on Powell's credentials and medical abilities continued.

On July 19, 1883, the *Morning Chronicle* reported that Alberta, Frank Powell's wife, had gone to the seaside for the summer. Six days later, George Powell's wife, Elizabeth, left La Crosse for an extended visit with her father in Montreal. It was evident that Powell's family was preparing for his ensuing defense against his critics.

On July 24, Powell began an assault against his detractors that continued for three days—paying the *Morning Chronicle* to run a series of articles that included his credentials. White Beaver's opening press salvo is illuminating: "Because I came to La Crosse a stranger, not satisfied to wallow in professional mire, a few of the doctors of this city have continually striven to do me harm by maliciously and deliberately lying about me. For two years I have remained silent, hoping that the fire of local medical malice would consume itself. Now I say to those who slandered me: Produce your diplomas! If any physician in this city can show as many honestly earned credentials as the undersigned I will give five

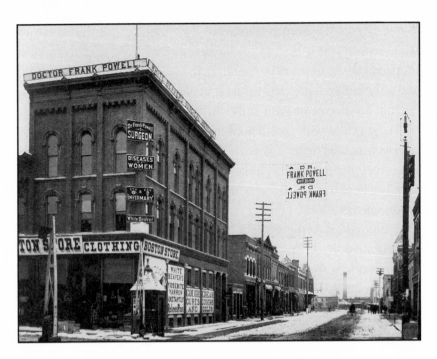

Dr. Frank Powell's offices in La Crosse, Wisconsin.
Photo courtesy Murphy Library, University of Wisconsin at La Crosse,
neg. no. 6783.

hundred dollars to the poor fund of this city. Put up or shut up." No one "put up or shut up."

A published offer on July 27 temporarily quieted Powell's opponents: "I hereby challenge any one of the doctors who have been traducing me to meet me in open debate.... Then if I cannot satisfy the audience assembled that I am as familiar with the gentleman's own theme as himself I promise to never practice my profession another day in the city of La Crosse." It is not surprising that there was no debate; some university-trained medical doctors of the era received their diplomas after only six weeks of classes and passing a test.

In addition to defending himself against his critics, Powell had to distinguish himself from impersonators and squelch false rumors about him. Dr. Diamond Dick, a specialist in "Indian Methods Alone" who resembled Powell, set up shop in La Crosse and soon was thrown in jail for assaulting a policeman. On January 24, 1884, Powell's agent ran an ad in the *Morning Chronicle* warning people about an individual impersonating Powell; in addition, Powell also had to set the record straight about lies circulating in Chippewa Falls about a nonexistent ne'er-do-well son-in-law.

However, none of these actions by the area's rival doctors intimidated White Beaver. Late in 1883 Powell decided to expand his medical practice into St. Paul. To legally practice in Minnesota, he needed to be certified by the newly created Minnesota Medical Examiners Board. What should have been a mere formality, however, became an opportunity for his competition to challenge him, and the medical board rejected his application.

As a result, Powell filed a writ of mandamus against the Minnesota medical board to force it to issue him a license for practicing medicine in the state. Not only did Powell prove that he had practiced medicine in Lanesboro, Minnesota, for more than four years—one possible way to be certified—he also sent the medical board his diploma, which it acknowledged as legitimate. After the *St. Paul Pioneer Press* printed a story on January 19, 1884, entitled "White Beaver—How the St. Paul Physicians Regard the Chances for Freezing Out the Winnebago Medicine Man," Powell took the offensive. On the front page of the January 23, 1884, issue of the *La Crosse Morning Chronicle* appeared a letter from Powell, informing the medical community that he would not be bluffed, and complaining that not only did he pay 50 cents a line for his back-page "news" articles but that "regular doctors" got articles printed for free. In addition, he said, he had worked for his education, unlike most "regular doctors."

On February 1, 1884, the *Morning Chronicle* stated that Powell had "backed down" the Minnesota state medical board. "They had tackled a man who is neither a quack, an incompetent, a coward nor a fool, and decided to keep their hands off." Throughout 1884, newspapers and private citizens supported Powell with testimonials, which Powell had published, and newspapers printed articles defending Powell's medical abilities and his advertising budget. James William Buell included a fanciful heroic biography of Powell in *Heroes of the Plains*, and Buffalo Bill featured White Beaver Powell in four dime novels. In those novels, the readers could supposedly expect "a rare treat where fact and fiction are combined." Cody also gave Powell a number of expensive gifts and purchased one-half interest in "White Beaver's Cough Cream" for $20,000.

In April 1884, the *Chicago Inter-Ocean* reported that a party of drunken Sioux attempted to assassinate Powell. The party may have been put up to it by detractors of White Beaver's because they hid the botched attempt with a concocted story that the assassins' leader's brother Yellow Hair had been killed by Dr. Powell and wanted revenge. During the 1876 Plains Wars, Bill Cody had killed a Yellow Hand, also known as Yellow Hair, but not Dr. Powell. At any rate, Powell had taken the pistol from the Indian, found the pistol did not work, and pistol-whipped the man into unconsciousness.

Despite the support of his medical practice from private citizens and the promotion of Powell by Cody and others, in July 1884 the Minnesota Supreme Court upheld the medical examining board's decision not to grant Powell a certificate to practice medicine because "in associating himself with the Winnebago tribe of Indians and accepting the name 'White Beaver, the Medicine Man' [he] had committed an unprofessional act." The *St. Paul Dispatch* stated, "The Supreme Court is getting down to a microscopic business in trying to construe that humbug enactment." Powell wrote the medical board that he would send them a disputed medicine formula for White Beaver's Cough Cream if they would send him an uncanceled two-cent stamp "less ⅛th for my Indian blood." Despite the state Supreme Court ruling, White Beaver kept his St. Paul offices open, and neither the police nor members of the medical board intervened.

In the face of this adversity, the Powell brothers, who had previously been only loosely associated, now closed ranks and occupied the same business apartments. An August 12, 1884, *Morning Chronicle* article that might have been written by White Beaver stated, "Coming here in the face of much prejudice among a certain class who derided the homeopathic quantity of Indian blood in their veins, they have by their square dealing and most wonderful success overcome all obstacles."

A major opportunity to silence the slander and enhance his reputation presented itself to Powell on March 21, 1885, when La Crosse Mayor William A. Roosevelt withdrew from an upcoming mayoral race and a "People's Convention," attended by Drs. Frank, George, and William Powell, started a draft movement to elect White Beaver to the mayor's office because "he has bravely withstood the assaults made upon him by the press and some of the medicine men of the city, and undoubtly [*sic*] attained great popularity, especially among the working people." Although Powell did not announce his candidacy until three days before the election on April 4, when the election was held on April 7 he won by a plurality of 252.

Following the election, the *Morning Chronicle* stated on several occasions that it did not support Powell, only ran his paid advertisements, and that Powell had no real powers as mayor. However, the *Morning Chronicle* had underestimated Powell, who immediately fired policeman William Duncan for "displaying an unbecoming partisan zeal to further personal desires and because he used scurrilous and malicious language when speaking of the chief executive."

A letter to the editor of the *Morning Chronicle* written by "An Independent Voter" had this to say:

> It only seems that the politicians reckoned on the election of the mayor with the doctor left out. The people appeared to think he ought not be left out and hence the "in-ness" of the doctor at the present time. He defeated the regular party nominees and that is the head and foot of his offending. Since it is so, why not swallow your mortification, gentlemen of the opposition, and give Dr. Powell a fair trial before you condemn him? The objection to the length of the doctor's hair is puerile and impertinent.... If people are disposed to call him an Indian we know that it is true, his connection with the "first families of America" is thereby firmly established and the know-nothings ought to be satisfied. The doctor certainly has more personal dignity than most of his detractors and is in no sense a man discreditable to La Crosse.

After the incident with Officer Duncan, the slanderous personal attacks on Powell ceased. White Beaver became the leader of the Populist movement in Wisconsin and ran for governor in 1888 and 1894. Newspaper editorials castigated White Beaver as a political demagogue, but after Powell won his heated four-year battle with the medical establishments in La Crosse and St. Paul, even White Beaver's detractors admitted that the "Medicine Chief of the Winnebagos" was a doctor of unquestioned skill. White Beaver and his "Winnebago vote" became a force that Wisconsin's political powerbrokers had to take into account until "the Beaver," as papers often called Powell, left Wisconsin in 1900 to oversee speculative western developments that he owned with Buffalo Bill. Frank Powell died in El Paso, Texas, on May 6, 1906, while on a train from Los Angeles.

Like his "blood brother" Buffalo Bill Cody, Powell could talk a good story and was a self-promoter. While both characters have received strong doses of criticism, both men actually provided valuable services. Buffalo Bill offered good entertainment; what his friend White Beaver provided was good medicine.

BIBLIOGRAPHIC ESSAY

This article first appeared in *Wild West,* October 1994. For the past decade I have lectured on, and appeared as, William F. Cody, a man who I deeply admire as a dreamer. After a performance of my solo show "Cody! An Evening with 'Buffalo Bill'" at the Grand Encampment Museum in Encampment, Wyoming, in the spring of 1990, I was informed that Bill Cody had owned a gold mine there with his "blood brother" Frank Powell. Very little had been written about Dr. Franklin David "White Beaver" Powell at that time, and much of it was poorly researched.

This gap in Cody scholarship motivated my search for the real Dr. Powell, which began at the Buffalo Bill Historical Center with my friend and mentor, Dr. Paul Fees, Senior Curator. There were a few articles in this collection about Powell, but, more importantly, Paul had a copy of Mary Hardgrove Hebbard's "Notes on Dr. David Frank Powell, Known as White Beaver," published in the *Wisconsin Magazine of History* (Summer 1952). Even though a lot of Hebbard's material on Powell is taken from James William Buell's apocryphal *Heroes of the Plains* (San Francisco, Calif.: A. L. Bancroft & Co., 1893), her comments and notes on Powell's medical practice led me to read the *La Crosse Morning Chronicle* and the *Republican and Leader.* The editors of both these newspapers had very definite opinions about Powell that became more newsworthy after Powell entered the political arena. Ellis Usher, the owner and editor of the *Morning Chronicle,* supported Powell until "the Beaver" contested him for political mastery of La Crosse in the 1890s, and William Rufus Finch, owner and editor of the *Republican and Leader,* hated the Powell brothers because they were "Injuns."

While checking the resources at the University of Wisconsin in La Crosse, I met Ed Hill, who is in charge of the Murphy Library Special Collection. He and his staff were very informative and supportive. They steered me to the Lanesboro (Minnesota) Historical Society, where I contacted Donald Ward, who possesses a treasure trove of information and newspaper clippings about Powell and Cody in Lanesboro. Another researcher I found helpful was Brigid Shields, reference librarian with the Minnesota Historical Society, who located the records on the Minnesota Supreme Court case of *Powell v. the Minnesota Medical Examining Board.* The racism in these legal documents is all too apparent.

To discover why the Minnesota Medical Examining Board and other doctors in the area objected to Powell and felt threatened by him, I did background research on medical practices at the turn of the century. Among other works, I consulted Gerald Carson's *One for a Man, Two for a Horse* (Garden City, N.Y.: Doubleday, 1961), a fine illustrated text on quack medicine that has a brief discussion about White Beaver's Cough Cream and Cody's endorsements for Kickapoo medicines. The more in-depth scholarly texts included these often amusing books: *The Golden Age of Quackery* by Stewart H. Holbrook (New York: Collier Books, 1962); *The Natural History of Quackery* by Eric Jameson (London: Michael Joseph, 1961); and *The Toadstool Millionaires* by James Harvey Young (Princeton, N.J.: Princeton University Press, 1961).

For actual medical texts of the period, I consulted these dry tomes: *Rheumatism, Gout, and Some Allied Disorders* by Morris Longstreth (New York: William Wood & Company, 1882) and *Applied Physiology* by Frank Overton (New York: American Book Company, 1897). Longstreth recommends the common practice of ingesting mercury to cure rheumatism, and Overton's text has some wonderful illustrations of medical devices of the era. For general contemporary medical texts, see: *The Household Physician* by A. T. Lovering (Boston: Woodruff Publishing Company, 1905); *The People's Common Sense Medical Adviser* by R. V. Pierce (Buffalo, N.Y.: The World's Dispensary Printing Office and Bindery, 1909); and *Medicology*, edited by James P. Wood (New York, Philadelphia, and London: University Medical Society, 1907).

I also talked with Dr. Sherrill Redmon, archivist for the University of Louisville, and Colleen Schiavone, project archivist, about the quality of medicine taught at the Louisville Medical College in the 1870s. They enlightened me about the college's course of instruction and informed me that medical students who followed different methodologies frequently fought duels. See *The History of the University of*

Louisville by Dwayne Cox (Louisville, Ky.: University of Louisville Archives, 1992).

Dime novels by Bill Cody bolstered Powell's reputation and rewrote his sordid military career, failed marriage, and official "blacklisting" by the surgeon general while Powell worked as a contract surgeon of the American plains. They contain tantalizing clues about Powell's first wife, who didn't leave her name for posterity. All written by William Frederick Cody, the novels include *White Beaver's Still Hunt; or The Miner Marauder's Death Track* (New York: Beadle & Adams, 1894); *White Beaver, the Exile of the Platte; or, A Wrong Man's Red Trail* (New York: Beadle & Adams, 1886); and *The Wizard Brothers; or, White Beaver's Red Trail* (New York: Beadle & Adams, 1886).

Other writers, friends of Cody's, found "White Beaver" and his brothers "Night Hawk" George and "Bronco Billie" to be characters worthy of being in over forty dime novels, such as the following titles by Colonel Prentiss Ingraham: *White Beaver, The Indian Medicine Chief; or, The Romantic & Adventurous Life of Dr. D. Frank Powell, Known on the Border as "Fancy Frank," "Iron Face," etc.* (New York: Beadle & Adams, 1884); *Bronco Billy, The Saddle Prince* (New York: Beadle & Adams, 1899); *Night-Hawk George, and His Daring Deed and Adventures in the Wilds of the South and West* (New York: Beadle & Adams, 1882).

Writing dime novels was not beneath Powell himself, who authored *Old Grizzly Adams, the Bear Tamer; or "The Monarch of the Mountains"* (New York: M. J. Ivers & Co., 1899) and *The Dragoon Detective; or a Man of Destiny* (New York: Beadle & Adams, 1893). For an overview of these titles, see *The House of Beadle and Adams and Its Dime and Nickel Novels Vol. I & II* by Albert Johannsen (Norman: University of Oklahoma Press, 1950).

I can recommend that people interested in Bill Cody limit their reading to the "bible" of Cody scholarship, *The Lives and Legends of Buffalo Bill* by Don Russell (Norman: University of Oklahoma Press, 1960).

Finally, I studied in numerous archives that held many undiscovered gems about Buffalo Bill's blood brother, Powell—the notorious "Injun" who defied the era's racism, aligning himself with the victors of the Little Big Horn, and led Wisconsin's Populist movement. Included in the archival material is information about the 1894 election in which White Beaver ran for governor of Wisconsin on the most radical egalitarian platform in the country.

William Kroeger: The "Priest-Healer" of Epiphany, South Dakota

JAMES MARTEN

On December 8, 1904, a young woman named Anton Herald died of consumption far from her Iowa home in a hotel in the South Dakota hamlet of Epiphany. The reputation of a local doctor named William Kroeger (1853–1904) had led her brother to take her there. Unfortunately for Herald and scores of other hopeful patients awaiting treatment at Kroeger's sanitarium, the fifty-one-year-old Kroeger had died that same winter day, ending his eleven-year medical career in South Dakota.

Kroeger had come to Epiphany in 1893 and by 1900 had earned something approaching national prominence. Perhaps four hundred patients came to his sanitarium, or laboratory, each week at the height of his business, and thousands of other clients sampled the products of Father Kroeger's Remedy Company. According to an article in the *Canova Herald* his dollar-per-flask patent medicine could cure "epileptic fits, St. Vitus Dance and Nervous Debility," as well as "St. Anthony's Dance, Nervousness, Kidney Troubles, Bowel Complaints and Womb Troubles." He also marketed a "Rheumatic Cure," a salve for "ulcerated limbs, open limbs, feet or hands," a cold, throat, and lungs formula, and potions for "catarrh of the stomach," blood disorders, and diarrhea.

A booming clinic complemented Kroeger's mail-order practice. Tubercular, cancerous, and otherwise sickly people flowed into Epiphany, where they received a variety of treatments in addition to Kroeger's liquid remedies. He trained his nurse, a twenty-seven-year-old German immigrant by the name of Louise Mentele, and his assistant, a former teacher and office clerk named Benjamin Ripperda, to administer ointments and compresses to "draw" cancers out of patients. In addition, by 1903 Kroeger had purchased three X-ray machines that he used to treat lung diseases and skin cancers. Stories of his success spread, and eager

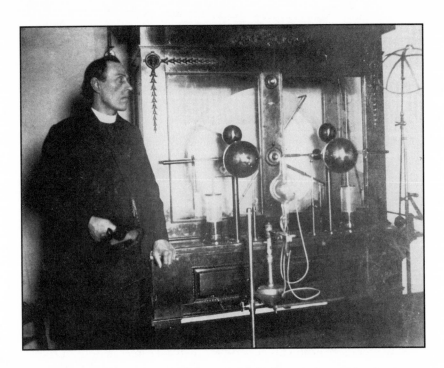

William Kroeger came to Epiphany, South Dakota, as the parish priest in
1893, but his ministrations soon shifted from the community's spiritual
concerns to its medical needs. The priest-healer, as Kroeger was known,
is shown here with his early X-ray machine.
Photo courtesy Sioux Falls Diocese Archives, Sioux Falls, South Dakota.

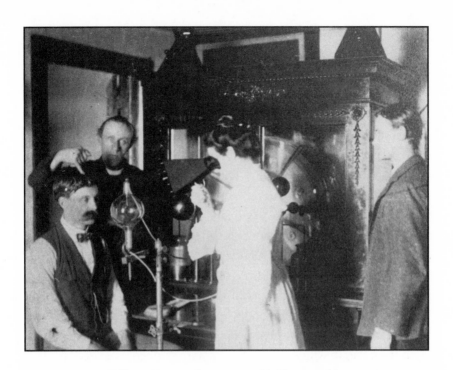

William Kroeger demonstrates his X-ray machine.
Photo courtesy Sioux Falls Diocese Archives, Sioux Falls, South Dakota.

health-seekers—whose numbers swelled tiny Epiphany to two or three times its regular size—filled private homes, hay mows, and vacant railroad cars waiting for their turn at the clinic.

On a typical day late in his career, Kroeger examined patients from 9 A.M. to noon—except on Sundays, some holidays, and during his three-month summer hiatus. At times, he scheduled as many as 130 people a day. Potential clients had to write to him in advance, telling him which day they would be in Epiphany. Then he would assign each of them a number corresponding to his or her place in line for that particular day. In spite of these restrictions, as many as 600 hopeful patients would sometimes crowd into Epiphany, the surrounding towns, and throughout the countryside, hoping for a few moments with the famed healer. Kroeger's mail and related business required the efforts of two stenographers, a private secretary, and a full-time bookkeeper.

Kroeger dominated the economy of his town. He not only produced his own medicines and treated his own patients, but he also manufactured the boxes in which the medicines were shipped, operated the dray lines that transported many of his patients from local railheads to Epiphany and the hotels in which they stayed, controlled the print shop that printed his advertisements and labels, ran his own water and electrical plants, published a short-lived newspaper—the *Kroeger Echo*—and owned the bank in which he deposited his money. Virtually everyone in town worked for Kroeger or depended on the business he brought in. Local girls served as waitresses and domestics in the town's three hotels, while homeowners and farmers could make $20 a night putting up would-be patients. Others made as much as $2.50 a day driving passengers to and from depots in neighboring towns like Canova and Spencer.

Kroeger's entrepreneurial medical career was unusual because it flourished in a tiny prairie backwater without its own rail service. It was even more unique because Kroeger had come to Epiphany in 1893 as the town's Roman Catholic priest. Born in Cincinnati in 1853 and an 1880 graduate of St. Meinrad, a Benedictine seminary in Indiana, Kroeger had served as priest at St. Vincent's Church in Elkhart, Indiana, for a dozen years before he moved to Epiphany—perhaps recruited by Reverend Martin Marty, the former abbot of St. Meinrad, whose diocese was strapped for qualified priests. To meet the needs of his far-flung parishioners—he had only sixty priests to administer to the 48,000 Catholics in South Dakota—the bishop accepted a number of what Marty's biographer, Robert Karolevitz, has called "malcontents, alcoholics and assorted trouble-makers."

According to reports, once he arrived in Epiphany Kroeger quickly got a new church built before Bishop Marty suggested Kroeger put his medical knowledge to good use in the poor, doctorless parish. However, as Kroeger's practice spread outside the immediate area, Marty's successor, Thomas O'Gorman, demanded that the so-called "priest-healer" choose one vocation or the other, citing church legislation that forbade priests from practicing medicine. The Vatican denied Kroeger's appeal in 1898, and eventually he was suspended from the priesthood.

While the Catholic Church obviously had very clear guidelines about the training and responsibilities of priests, Kroeger's medical profession had far less precise regulations in that era. At various times, Kroeger named three different Ohio medical schools as his alma mater—but he had never attended two of them, and the third did not exist. Aside from the obvious ethical implications, the presence or absence of a diploma from a bona fide medical school was irrelevant during those years. Scores of turn-of-the-century mail-order doctors and even legitimate physicians practiced their own brands of medicine perfectly legally without medical degrees or professional memberships. In fact, in 1900 the fifty-four-year-old American Medical Association still carried less than one-fourth of the nation's 33,000 physicians on its rolls.

Adding to the mystery of Kroeger's life are the two years that passed between his departure from St. Vincent's in Elkhart and his arrival in South Dakota. There is some evidence to suggest that he had run up large financial debts in Indiana, where he had operated a dray line, grocery store, and patent medicine company when he was not running his parish. After his death, the *Alexandria Herald*'s obituary mentioned admiringly that Kroeger had paid off $40,000 in debts, adding tantalizingly that "while his life has not been blameless, he was his own worse enemy."

It is possible that Kroeger found inspiration for his own medical career in the exploits of two fellow Elkhart residents who made fortunes in the patent medicine business. From the 1850s through the 1880s, A. N. Chamberlain sold a Green Mountain Salve said to cure diarrhea,

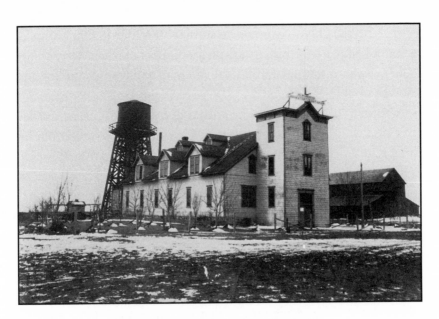

William Kroeger's laboratory and sanitarium.
Photo courtesy Sioux Falls Diocese Archives, Sioux Falls, South Dakota.

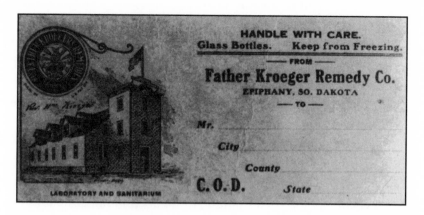

Shipping label for Father Kroeger Remedy Co.
Photo courtesy Sioux Falls Diocese Archives, Sioux Falls, South Dakota.

catarrh, colic in horses, sprains, neuralgia, toothache, and cholera. Dr. Charles F. Miles's Restorative Nervine, which the *Elkhart Sentinel* called a "brain and nerve food," earned a national reputation—and notoriety among muckraking journalists after 1900—for curing headaches, nervousness, spasms, sleeplessness, and sexual weakness. Perhaps even more inspirational to the young priest were the potential profits to be made; by 1900, the industry did $30,000,000 a year.

Although Louise Mentele's niece suggested many years after Kroeger's death that the recipe for at least one of the doctor's cures had actually been brought from Germany by Mentele's father, Kroeger was the entrepreneur who profited from the formula. Testimonials published in the *Canova Herald*—like the remarkably similar-sounding testimonials from other medicines—attested to his skill and to the efficacy of his concoctions. One correspondent reported that the epileptic fits that had tormented him for thirty years had vanished. Another claimed that he had wasted $400 on operations to rid his son of "stagnation of the nerves." After the application of one of the priest's medicines, however, the boy ran "around and [played] with the other children as if nothing had ailed him."

Articles published in faraway newspapers such as the *St. Paul Dispatch* promised that Kroeger needed no more than three weeks to cure cancer and consumption. By 1903, according to Doane Robinson's *History of South Dakota*, patients flocked to the sanitarium "from every state of the Union and all over the world." Railroad companies added special cars for patients heading for Epiphany; occasionally Sioux Indians would come over from their reservations west of the Missouri River.

Kroeger's greatest claim to medical innovation was his extensive use of X-ray therapy. Discovered in late 1895 by Wilhelm Conrad Röntgen, X-rays promptly seized the imagination of Americans when word of their discovery reached the United States a few months later. Credulous readers of newspapers and scientific periodicals learned that the rays could project anatomical diagrams directly into the brains of medical students, eliminate the need for surgery, transform metal into gold, cure alcoholism, and help spiritualists by photographing thought processes. Physicians and technicians immediately began looking for medical applications for the new technology. Initial ideas for utilizing X-rays included the now-familiar techniques of locating bone fractures, foreign bodies, signs of arthritis and sarcomas, and orthopedic oddities, but other researchers—driven by more entrepreneurial visions than by medical common sense—insisted that the cumbersome X-ray machines could be used to kill pain, treat tuberculosis, and reduce cancers of the skin, bone, lip, and breast. Although the high cost and the serious side effects of the treatment discouraged many practitioners, incredibly, cancer patients submitted to two thirty-minute sessions every day for a week. Not surprisingly, the treatment caused nausea, blisters, hair loss, and inflamed eyes. As a result, most doctors and hospitals refused to use X-rays routinely until well into the 1910s or 1920s.

But not William Kroeger. As early as 1900 he had installed three machines in his laboratory, which were primarily used to treat cancer. Since X-ray therapy temporarily reduced pain and did, in some cases, eliminate less severe sarcomas, Kroeger gained a reputation as an expert in treating one of the most feared and mysterious conditions of the late nineteenth century. Doctors had searched in vain for a cause of the "dread disease," having considered whether germs caused it, or heredity, or disharmony between humans and their environment as a result of industrialization, or emotional or mental stress, or even illicit sex. Cancer treatments were frequently painful and rarely effective; exploiting the public's fear and loathing, physicians like Kroeger produced tonics, caustic pastes or poultices, and elaborate electrical apparatuses to "cure" cancer. Kroeger made X-ray therapy the centerpiece of his fight against cancer. Evidence suggests that the three machines in Epiphany were in constant operation several hours a day, including Saturdays. A 1904 notice in the *Kroeger Echo* emphasized that prospective patients who wanted to be X-rayed needed to provide Kroeger with advance notice and that "all that have corset[s] on must remove them." Ironically, it is not unlikely that Kroeger's untimely death was due to exposure to X-rays rather than the dropsy mentioned in contemporary obituaries.

Kroeger's reputation as a cancer specialist and his shrewd business dealings made him a wealthy man. In August 1900, the *Mitchell Daily Republican* reported that he had "made a mint of money since he commenced to practice medicine." At the time of his death, the *Alexandria Herald* reported that he left a "vast fortune." Estimates ranged from $175,000 to $250,000. Evidence of his healthy finances came when Kroeger began taking summers off during the last several years of his career, often traveling to Europe or the Holy Land, sometimes accompanied by Mentele.

When Kroeger returned from a trip to Europe in October 1904, it was clear that his health had failed, and although the public believed his illness was not life-threatening, Kroeger apparently suspected differently. He successfully petitioned the bishop for absolution and reinstatement, saying mass one last time before dying on December 8, 1904. Nine priests and a large crowd of admirers attended his funeral three days later. Buried in the cemetery of the church to which he had come only eleven years before, he now lies under an imposing stone cross.

Neither his business enterprises nor the prosperity of Epiphany survived Kroeger's death. His demise, declared the *Canova Herald*, "means a loss to Epiphany from which the town can scarcely recover." Three weeks after his death, the town "present[ed] a true aspect of mourning for its founder." The laboratory was closed, and the electric lights were turned off. A month later, John Krempges, the druggist who actually mixed the secret remedies in Kroeger's laboratory, left to study chemistry at the state college in Brookings. In mid-March, Kroeger's *Echo* stopped publishing. Despite Kroeger's wishes that his work be carried on after his death, Mentele failed to convince the State Board of Medical Examiners, with whom she met in late January, to allow her to continue the practice. In late February, she announced that Kroeger's assets would be sold at auction. Someone—it is unclear who—continued producing and selling bottled remedies under the name of the Father Kroeger Remedy Company for perhaps a decade, but even that end of the business ultimately failed to survive. Eventually the buildings were torn down or collapsed, although descendants of Mentele lived in one of the town's hotels, complete with faded room numbers on the doors, into the 1970s.

Kroeger's life and career pose several paradoxes. An enthusiastic priest, his commitment to the Catholic Church nevertheless took a back seat to his medical practice. Although on his deathbed he sought and received the restoration of his rights as a priest, he left the bulk of his sizeable estate to his friend and partner Louise Mentele, rather than to his church or any other charitable enterprise. He was a hardworking medical man and apparently dedicated to his patients; however, rather than following the difficult path of scientific investigation and innovation—the course followed by his contemporaries, the Mayo brothers, who worked a few hundred miles to the east in southeastern Minnesota—he focused on easy answers and shadowy miracle cures even as he took advantage of twentieth-century technologies. Although he was not the saint that many of his contemporaries believed him to be, he was probably not the questionable character that some elements of his life (the misrepresentation of his medical school background and his undefined relationship with Louise Mentele, for example) might indicate. The most accurate, though perhaps the least satisfying, solution to the puzzle that was Kroeger is simply to view him as a man of his times. Taking advantage of traditional beliefs and practices, existing conditions, and modern developments, Kroeger carved a niche for himself in the turn-of-the-century West.

BIBLIOGRAPHIC ESSAY

An earlier version of this article appeared in *South Dakota History* 21, no. 4 (1991). Copyright 1991 by the South Dakota State Historical Society. All rights reserved. Reprinted by permission.

Much of the information on William Kroeger comes from newspapers published in towns near Epiphany, including the *Mitchell Daily Republic,* the *Canova Herald,* and the *Alexandria Journal* and *Herald.* Files of the *Echo* have not survived, although the papers previously mentioned occasionally copied articles from the priest's "official" newspaper.

Other useful primary sources include files and photographs located in the archives of the Catholic Chancery Office of the Diocese of Sioux Falls, South Dakota, and the Margaret Mentele interview from the Dakota State College Oral History Project (housed at the South Dakota State Historical Society).

An informative account of South Dakota Catholicism—including information about Kroeger—is Robert F. Karolevitz's *With Faith, Hope and Tenacity: The First One Hundred Years of the Catholic Diocese of Sioux Falls, 1889–1989* (Mission Hill, S.D.: Dakota Homestead Publishers, 1989). The original source for many of the brief articles published about Kroeger since the early 1950s has apparently been Doane Robinson's *History of South Dakota,* 2 vols. (n.p.: B.F. Bowen & Co., 1904). Written while Kroeger was still alive, it includes short biographies and photographs of the doctor and his assistants, and presents a number of myths regarding his career.

Providing context for Kroeger's story were a number of secondary works: John H. Warner, *The Therapeutic Perspective: Medical Practice, Knowledge, and Identity in America, 1820–1885* (Cambridge, Mass.: Harvard University Press, 1986); Paul Starr, *The Social Transformation of American Medicine* (New York: Basic Books, 1982); Stewart H. Holbrook, *The Golden Age of Quackery* (New York: Macmillan, 1959); James Harvey Young, *The Toadstool Millionaires: A Social History of Patent Medicines in America Before Federal Regulation* (Princeton, N.J.: Princeton University Press, 1961); James T. Patterson, *The Dread Disease: Cancer and Modern American Culture* (Cambridge, Mass.: Harvard University Press, 1987); and Otto Glasser, *Wilhelm Röntgen and the Early History of the Röntgen Rays* (Springfield, Ill.: Charles C. Thomas, 1934).

Daring Dr. Sofie

CINDI MYERS

When word spread that a new doctor was arriving in the frontier town of Brazoria, Texas, in 1893, many people were shocked to learn the physician was a woman. Further investigation would have revealed that she was a widow with fourteen grown children, and that she was moving to Texas all the way from New York City. What kind of a woman was she?

Anyone who awaited Dr. Sofie Herzog's arrival expecting some grandmotherly midwife must have been dumbfounded at the attractive, energetic, and highly skilled physician who confronted them. Only forty-five years old, Herzog (1848–1925) was a graduate of a Vienna, Austria, university, where she had trained with some of the most prestigious physicians of the day. She had managed a successful medical practice in New York but went to Texas for the same reason many other people did—adventure.

Thick woods, palmetto marshes, and overgrown fields comprised the Brazos River bottomlands in the 1890s and offered outlaws plenty of hiding places. In Brazoria, men continued to settle their arguments with fists and guns, and a poor economy, short tempers, and Texas heat produced more than one nasty gun battle. Natural enemies ranging from alligators and rattlesnakes to malaria and yellow fever also took their toll on the populace. In a place that needed a brave physician, Herzog found her home.

In that era, physicians were still a rarity in that part of the country, and female or not, "Dr. Sofie," as she became known, had little trouble establishing her medical practice. She quickly impressed—and at times astounded—her patients with her medical skill and seeming disregard for conventions of the day.

At a time when fashion dictated that women wear their hair long and coiled atop their heads, Dr. Sofie cut her brown curls short. After discovering that muddy streets made buggy travel difficult, she bought a

165

horse and had a local seamstress make her a divided skirt. Thereafter people often saw her riding through town astride her horse, a man's hat shoved down over her short hair, hurrying to the next patient.

Among other skills, Dr. Sofie quickly earned a reputation for removing bullets. She so delighted in the compliments she received for this skill that she had a necklace made of bullets she removed from patients, with a gold bead threaded through each slug. The necklace eventually had twenty-four bullets, and Dr. Sofie wore the unique piece of jewelry often, claiming it brought her luck. The really lucky individuals, however, were the patients under Dr. Sofie's care.

Dr. Sofie was born in Austria in 1848; her father was an internationally-known surgeon. She was only fourteen when she married her husband, who was also a surgeon, and in twenty-six years of marriage the couple had fourteen children, including two sets of twins. Despite her many family responsibilities, caring for her large family was not enough for Dr. Sofie. She studied medicine in order to help her husband and continued to assist him when he moved his practice to New York in 1886.

The Herzogs had been in the United States only a few years when Dr. Sofie's husband died. She continued to practice medicine in New York until 1893, when she decided to follow her youngest daughter, Elfriede Marie, and her husband, Randolph Prell, to Texas.

At the time medicine was not a profession for the fainthearted. Among the instruments considered essential for any doctor were a saw for amputations and pliers for extracting teeth. Doctors had no antibiotics and few pain-killers besides whiskey and, occasionally, morphine. Bloodletting continued as an established medical procedure until late in the nineteenth century, and Dr. Sofie's black bag would certainly have contained a lancet for producing puncture wounds to release blood. Doctors of the time also used leeches to draw blood, although special medicinal leeches were preferable to those Dr. Sofie could have found in the local streams.

Tonics and patent medicines were very popular, and pitchmen widely advertised their fantastic claims. Many people relied on home remedies for common illnesses and accidents and called a doctor only as a last resort. Physicians like Dr. Sofie depended on quinine, calomel, mustard plasters, and castor oil to treat most ailments, and they relied heavily on their own knowledge and common sense.

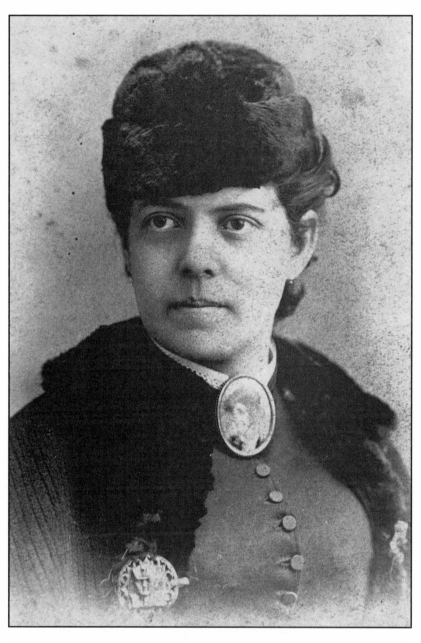

Trained in Vienna, Dr. Sofie Herzog came to Brazoria, Texas, from New York City in 1893. When she died in 1925, after a long and successful practice, she was buried wearing a necklace made of bullets that she had removed from patients.
Photo courtesy Archives Division, Texas State Library, neg. no. 1975/70-5431.

Dr. Sofie lived with the Prells when she first arrived in Brazoria, and she practiced out of their house. But her interest in treating all types of medical cases did not lead to family harmony. She once smuggled a smallpox patient into the house, intending to try out a new ointment she had developed to treat the disease. Her son-in-law heard what she had done and burst into the room as she was applying the ointment to the patient's back. The patient took one look at Prell's furious expression and fled. Dr. Sofie's son-in-law forbid her to ever bring a victim of such a horrible, contagious, and, at the time, much-feared disease into his home. After a long, loud argument, Dr. Sofie decided to build her own office, where she could treat patients and experiment with new methods uninterrupted. Subsequently, she had a three-room office built on Market Street, with living quarters in the back. Her son-in-law worried about her living alone and offered her a gun, but she refused the weapon.

Even without a gun, Dr. Sofie was apparently quite capable of looking after herself. According to one story, when a visitor gave her trouble and refused to leave her office, Dr. Sofie grabbed a poker from the fireplace and banished him.

"I want no odds because I'm a woman," Dr. Sofie once said—as quoted by Marie Beth Jones in *Brazosport Facts*—and indeed, it seems her gender never prevented her from doing what she wanted. In 1905, when construction began on the St. Louis, Brownsville and Mexico Railroad, Dr. Sofie applied for the post of railroad chief surgeon. Because she had already treated many of the railroad's workers and her former patients praised her abilities, she had little trouble getting the job.

However, evidently the railroad officials had no idea that the new company doctor who had been hired was a woman. After learning that startling news, they promptly asked Dr. Sofie to resign, but she declined.

"I'll keep this job so long as I give satisfaction," Dr. Sofie replied. The matter ended there, and she held the job for thirty years. Throughout her long career, Dr. Sofie repeatedly proved her abilities, traveling by horseback, boxcar, engine, or handcar to reach her patients along the railroad line. Her business cards, engraved in ornate letters, bore the inscription, "Local Surgeon, St. Louis, Brownsville and Mexico Railroad Company."

Once after securing the railroad job, Dr. Sofie was at a party with friends and barely escaped injury when a bullet tore through the door inches from her head. A local woman who wrongly thought Dr. Sofie had caused her husband to lose his job with the railroad had fired the shot. While others around her panicked, Dr. Sofie maintained her characteristic calm and shrugged off the incident.

Though she lived a rugged lifestyle and competed in a masculine world, Dr. Sofie never let it be forgotten she was a woman. She remained close to her fourteen children and loved to talk about her grandchildren. Moreover, she enjoyed needlework and kept a basket of it in her office so that she could sew or crochet in her free time.

But needlework would not have been the first thing visitors noticed when visiting Dr. Sofie's office. She decorated the small building with many wild animal skins, stuffed animal specimens, a collection of walking sticks, and medical specimens, including several premature or stillborn babies (one with two heads and three arms) preserved in jars of formaldehyde. After Dr. Sofie died, her granddaughter, Mrs. Henry Harang, had the specimens of babies buried. The other specimens were donated to the University of Texas Medical School at John Sealy Hospital in Galveston.

The Brazos River bottoms were a haven for rattlesnakes, and Dr. Sofie added many rattler skins to her animal skin collections. In addition, locals frequently brought dead snakes to her, which she hung on the side of her buggy house, skinned herself, and mounted on wide red ribbons to decorate her office walls. When Dr. Sofie expressed a desire for an alligator to add to her collection, a townsman delivered one to her office. Unfortunately, the beast was still alive. After lying stunned on the floor for a few moments, the animal began thrashing about—forcing Dr. Sofie to defend herself with her trusty poker.

In addition to her own office, Dr. Sofie built two other buildings in town. After a disagreement with the local Catholic church over maintenance of their little cemetery, Dr. Sofie joined her daughter and son-in-law in the Episcopalian congregation and financed the construction of a new church. She also built the Southern Hotel, a two-and-a-half-story edifice that provided lodging for visitors and served as the site of many balls and meetings.

Ever the trendsetter, Dr. Sofie was one of the first people in Brazoria to purchase an automobile. She took driving lessons from the salesman and soon began making her rounds behind the wheel of a Ford runabout.

At sixty-five, Dr. Sofie married for the second time. Her groom was Colonel Martin Huntington, five years her senior. But neither marriage nor age could stop Dr. Sofie; she continued to practice medicine for the rest of her life.

By the time Dr. Sofie died in July 1925, the rough-and-tumble town of Brazoria had shed most of its wilder ways. Dr. Sofie had seen many significant changes in her thirty-two years there, but she never forgot her early adventures. At her request, she was buried with her "good luck" bullet necklace.

BIBLIOGRAPHIC ESSAY

Works consulted include several articles by Marie Beth Jones from *Brazosport Facts* (1961): "Dr. Sofie Followed Daughter to Texas," January 18; "Bullet Necklace a 'Lucky Piece,'" January 25; "Dr. Sofie Was Railroad Doctor," February 1; "Office Exhibit a Bit Startling," February 8; "Dr. Sofie Builds a Church," February 16; "Sofie Combined Career, Family," February 22.

Ellen N. Murry wrote about Dr. Sofie in "Racking Chills and Fever" in *Star of the Republic Museum Notes* 13, no. 2 (Washington, Tex.: Star of the Republic Museum, winter 1988). Mrs. George Plunkett Red included Dr. Sofie in *The Medicine Man in Texas* (Houston, Tex.: Standard Printing and Lithographing Co., 1939). The chapter, "Sofie Herzog: Daring Doctor of Brazoria," appeared in *We Can Fly: Stories of Katherine Stinson and Other Gutsy Texas Women* by Mary Beth Rogers, Sherry A. Smith, and Janelle D. Scott (Austin: The Texas Foundation for Women's Resources, 1983).

Appendix A:
Excerpts from
The Indian Household Medicine Guide

BY J. I LIGHTHALL

Medicine. Medicine is not a humbug. The humbug is in its improper administration. When medicine is properly administered it comes to the sufferer as a gift from God. Medicine is unjustly judged. It is not medicine that is at fault, but it is those who give it without the proper knowledge of its effects, and when it is indicated. Medicine, when it is not properly given, proves an actual poison to the system. The Indian Materia Medica treats of herbs and vegetation in general. That is, that part of vegetation which is known by them to have medicinal properties. They will never injure the system when conformed to according to directions given. I will now invite your attention to our Materia Medica.

Gentiana. Gentian. The root is the medical part, and upon chewing it gives a very bitter taste. It is a plant that grows in the mountains of the Oriental countries. The crushed root can be obtained from almost any of our drug stores. It is found in the Southern and Middle States.

Medical properties and uses. Gentian is a splendid tonic to invigorate the stomach to active digestion, acts very favorably in all cases where there is scrofula and humors in the blood. It proves a very good substitute for tobacco, for those who are breaking themselves of the habit. As a tonic, fill a pint-bottle half full of the root, add half alcohol and half water, and after fourteen days standing it is ready for use. The dose is a teaspoonful before each meal. This will ward off chills and fever, or ague. I have known it to break chills where quinine had failed. Gentian can be truly called a tonic of the first class.

171

Arum Triphyllum. Indian Turnip. This is a very valuable remedy for hoarseness and loss of voice, and wherever there is a burning sensation and constriction of the throat, and when there is a thin glary discharge from the nose. It is a plant that grows generally throughout the middle states, and school boys have enough knowledge of its properties in a green state not to bite it when invited by his fellow playmate. It is a very valuable remedy when properly used.

It is, in its recent state, a powerful local irritant, and should be handled with care. The manner in which it should be taken is as follows:

Take one part of the pulverized turnip dried, and mix it with three parts of pulverized sugar—the sugar being of a granulated or loaf sugar character. Mix well; let it stand for twelve hours and then stir again, and in twelve hours it is ready for use. The dose is a pinch as large as a pea or bean every three or four hours for hoarseness, sore throat and ulceration.

Macrotys Racemosa. Black Cohosh. Rattle Root. Rattle Root is one of the finest remedies known in the Indian and Eclectic practice. Its medical powers and actions on the human system are simply wonderful. I have used it in over two thousand cases in which it was indicated, and it gave myself and the patients satisfaction. It grows in most parts of the United States. It has a long stalk that grows into several branches, and each branch has a long plume-like cluster of little round pods, which are full of seeds. When the stalk is shaken the seeds will rattle, producing a sound like that of a rattlesnake, from which it takes the name of rattle root. The root is the medicinal part, and is best gathered during the months of July, August, and September. The main body of the root should be cut into several pieces carefully, as you will find it full of dirt, and then dried, watching that it does not mold before it dries out.

Medical properties and uses. Without this plant or root the Indian squaw-doctor or midwife would feel that she had lost her king of female remedies. It is called by the Indians, squaw root. It is a very active remedy, in its proper administration, on the serous and mucous tissues, and for many cases of rheumatism, especially that of a muscular character. It acts on the nerves, and quiets nervous excitability. The Indian squaw doctors have their patients take this remedy two or three months before confinement, and it has that marked effect on them that they are never troubled with false rheumatic pains, hemorrhages, or lengthy labors. An Indian squaw, when following her tribe, if confined, will stop by the wayside for that day and wait upon herself, and the next day will proceed and overtake her tribe, while but few of our civilized women can get out of bed under the ninth or fourteenth day, and even after that they have to use strict care for a month or six weeks, and even longer. I know of no remedy that is better to overcome suppressed menstruation, or in words that are understood by all, the checked monthly flow, when it is caused by cold or nervous weakness. It is one of our very best remedies in a great many womb troubles. Girls, at the age of twelve, thirteen, or fourteen years, the time they usually enter womanhood, or the time when their monthlies become established, have often serious trouble with irregularity of flows; some flowing to a great extent, some not enough. In such cases as these this remedy is almost a certain relief, and cures if properly given. I prepare my tincture in this manner: Take the fine crushed root and fill a pint or quart bottle half full; keep it well corked, and shake once or twice every day for fourteen days. In female troubles I give from five to ten drops of the tincture in a teaspoonful of water four times a day. The largest dose should never exceed thirty drops; the smallest is one. In the treatment of rheumatism it is always better to combine the tincture of Prickly Ash with it in equal portions.

Symplocarpus Foetidus. Skunk Cabbage. This is a plant that may be known in particular by its smell, resembling a disturbed skunk. It is a very common plant, and should have more special medical attention than what it has had. I have found it a very valuable remedy in several cases.

Medical properties and uses. Skunk Cabbage is a splendid thing for hoarseness and sore throat, taken internally and used as a gargle. It is good in all cases of consumption where there is nervous irritation of the windpipe and bronchial tubes. It is good for irritability of the general nervous system. Dose, from 5 to 15 drops every two or three hours. The roots are the parts that are to be used. When you wish to dry them they should be separated into small bunches, for they are in such large clusters that they will mold near the center before they are dry.

August Flower. This is a weed that usually grows along creeks, and in sandy and rocky places. It has a yellow flower that blooms in the month of August, and the leaves and flowers should be gathered during that month. They have a very important medicinal property, beyond any physician's idea, and no doctor will be convinced of the fact until he has given it a fair trial.

Medical properties and uses. This plant, if not known in any other way, I am sure is known by the name of Dr. Green's August Flower, the great dyspeptic remedy. I am well acquainted with an old and eminent physician in Felicity, Ohio, formerly from Tennessee, where he practiced for the southern planters. His name is Dr. Gibson. He is a noted Eclectic, a gentleman and a scholar, a natural and practical herbalist, and has given the August Flower and its medical properties close and thorough attention, and values it very highly as a remedy for irritation of the mucous membrane [*sic*] of the stomach and bowels, kidneys and bladder. I knew of one case of a little boy about ten years of age, who had what many physicians would call indigestion. The boy complained of his stomach and bowels, and everything that he ate passed through him nearly in the same condition that he swallowed it. The attending physician brought all his knowledge to act on the case, and tried all that in his judgment was calculated to help or relieve the pathological condition. The remedies simply checked the trouble, but on quitting them it returned as bad as before. So the patient fell into the hands of Dr. Gibson, of Felicity, Ohio. He gave his medicine, and the boy quickly recovered. It was a mystery to me, and I, knowing the doctor to be a gentleman, and free to impart his valuable knowledge to all that he thought would use it for the good of suffering humanity, asked him what he gave the boy. He told me he gave him August Flower Pills of his own make, and in two days the boy was well and had natural discharges from his bowels, which was evidence to me that there is wonderful medical virtue in the August Flower, no matter who may ignore it. The August Flower acted as a mucous film to protect and soothe the irritated mucous membrane from the food, which, when the stomach and bowels were in that condition, proved an irritant instead of a strengthener and support. It acts kindly on the kidneys and liver. Good for dyspepsia and biliousness.

Take the leaves and tops of the plant, cut up fine and make a tincture. Dose, a teaspoonful three or four times a day. Or boil them down in a thick syrup, and take equal parts of gum arabic and flour and make into pills the size of a buck shot. Dose, from four to six per day, as the case may demand.

Verbascum Thapsus. Mullein. This is a very common plant, growing almost everywhere. The leaves and tops are the medicinal parts, and it is best used in [the] form of a hot tea or syrup.

Medical properties and uses. This remedy is very mild in its action, yet quite certain. It makes a very valuable cough syrup, quiets nervous excitation, and therefore induces sleep. For bad colds the hot tea should be drank [*sic*] on going to bed.

Podophyllin. May Apple. This plant grows in little armies, and bears a little yellow apple, called a May apple. The root has a powerful medical property called podophyllin. It was discovered by John King, M.D., Professor of Obstetrics in the Cincinnati Eclectic Medical Institute, and since its discovery it has become a noted remedy all over the medical world.

Medical properties and uses. This is a powerful hydrogogue cathartic, in large doses producing copious watery discharges from the bowels. It is a fine remedy when properly given, for torpid liver, or, in other words, liver complaint. It arouses the general secretions, and when given in large doses it is a powerful emetic as well as cathartic, relieving the stomach of all the bile and mucus that may be in it. It has in the past been given in entirely too large doses, but at the present it is given properly. The pills can be procured from all druggists. The half grains are the best. Dose, from one to two.

Verbena Hastata. Vervain. This is a very valuable plant. The root is the part we use in medicine. It should be dug in July or August.

Medical properties and uses. Vervain is a fine tonic, in small doses, to follow all forms of fever with during convalescence. In large doses it is an emetic, but should never be taken to that extent. It is a very valuable bitter tonic. To prepare it for bitters, fill a bottle half full of finely-chopped root, and then fill with good whisky. Dose, a teaspoonful three times a day. The root is best when green.

Humulus Lupulus. Hops. This is a plant that grows in the shape of a vine both in Europe and in the United States, along the hedges and old stumps and walls, and is cultivated and grown at the present time for its valuable properties. It is largely used in the brewing of ale, beer and porter, and is what might be termed one of the standard herbs. We certainly cannot value this gift of God to man in the line of a natural product too highly.

Medical properties and uses. Lupuline, or hops, is a mild sleep producer, and is quieting to the nervous system in a great many cases. A man was once cured of dyspepsia by drinking lager beer, and he afterwards found it was the hops in the beer that did the work. They are valuable in the form of a hot poultice applied to the parts affected with cramps or painful conditions. No family should be without hops in the house, or where they can readily obtain them. They will relieve cramps and pains of the womb, when put on the belly in a sack in a hot condition.

Stramonium. Jamestown Weed, or Jimson. This is a highly important remedy, and every doctor has use for it. If it were an article that cost as much as quinine everybody would think more of it, but, as it grows as free as the water flows it has been ignored and discredited by many, or to say the least, sadly neglected by the medical profession.

Medical properties and uses. The leaves, saturated in saltpetre [*sic*], dried, mashed up fine, and mixed with tobacco and smoked, will give almost instant relief to asthma or phthisic, or difficult breathing. Take the tops and leaves and boil to a thick syrup and mix with mutton tallow. This forms a fine pile ointment, to use on the parts after each evacuation. A hot poultice of the leaves will overcome cramps, nervousness, and produce sleep. It has been used internally with success in delirium tremens, but should only be given by a physician.

Artemisia Absenthium. Wormwood. I shall simply speak of its most important medical property, and that is, its power of destroying worms. I value it above all remedies that are noted for the power of expelling worms. Santonin is made from wormwood, and is the best worm medicine in the world. It is a powerful stimulant to the brain and nerve centers. It acts on the optic nerves and makes things look yellow.

Medical properties and uses. It is what I would term strictly a specific for worms. I have given it to children as much as three hundred times, and in only one case did it fail to expel worms. A brother homeopath of Augusta, Ky., gave the child worm medicine afterwards, and the child passed several worms. I always combine the santonin with senna or jalap. I will give you the recipe or prescription that will suit a child from three to ten years old.

Jalap, 5 grains; Senna, 10 grains; Santonin, 3 grains.

Mix and make in 3 powders, and give one every two hours, and in one hour from the last powder follow with oil. Dissolve each powder in sweetened water.

Sarsaparilla. This is a plant that grows in the shape of a vine, clambering stumps and stubs of trees, fences, and stone walls, in a majority of districts of the United States. The root is usually about one quarter of an inch in diameter, and is many feet and yards long, so that when you dig an entire root up without breaking it, you may truly call it a vegetable cord grown by nature, of a bright golden yellow color. The root is the part that we use, and should be gathered in the months of July and September. It is better to prepare it immediately after digging, but it will retain its virtues a number of months after digging. This root is one of our most valuable remedies, and of great value to the medical profession. Physicians have praised it through every classical publication in the land. Sarsaparilla is a remedy that is undoubtedly alterative in its action. It can be taken freely in the form of an infusion or decoction without fear of doing harm. To make a tincture of it, fill a bottle half full of the finely cut root, add equal parts of water and alcohol, and let stand fourteen days, shake well each day. Dose, a tablespoonful four or five times a day. In all bad cases of blood diseases and eruptions of the skin, a half pint of the strong tea of the root should be taken in connection with the tincture every day. Let the patient bathe the whole body twice a week with pure water, rubbing the skin after bathing well with a rough towel. Do not charge your stomach with nuts, knick knacks, and fat meats, and you will find, inside of four weeks, that sarsaparilla is a blood purifier and alterative. I saw a case of scrofula caused by bad vaccine virus. The flesh seemed as though it would fall from the bones, and the physicians that were in attendance gave her up and said she would have to die. The mother made a strong syrup or tea of sarsaparilla root and made her drink it instead of water. It did the work. She got well.

It has been used by millions, and has been recommended by the same number to be a very valuable remedy, and a remedy that should find a place in every house in the land.

Medical properties and uses. The medical properties of this plant is [*sic*] generally known as an alterative and blood purifier. It is noted in its blood purifying history. I have known of a number of cases of blood diseases that the common syrup of sarsaparilla has cured where noted physicians have failed in their attempts with their lauded remedies. It acts kindly and freely on the kidneys, gently stimulating the sudoriferous glands as well as the sebaceous glands of the skin. It increases the appetite, and gently counteracts a constipated condition of the bowels. When taken freely for a considerable length of time it will overcome and cure a majority of our many troublesome skin and scrofulous diseases. When a person takes it freely they will find it will act on the kidneys similar to watermelon, and the sweat from the skin will be of a greasy, waxy nature. Try it if you don't believe it.

Laurus Sassafras. Sassafras. This is a very fine aromatic bush and tree. I have seen large fields of the bush no taller than the common Indian cornstalk, and I have seen the bush in its adult age or growth as tall as the gigantic oak. The bark of the root is the part used in medicine and domestic use. The Indians of many tribes dig it and use it as a tea. If it were used by civilization instead of store tea and coffee, the stomach and digestion of civilization would be much better, and the owner more happy and hopeful.

Medical properties and uses. Sassafras is something used by a great many physicians, if for nothing more than merely to make their medicines pleasant and palatable for their patients to take. It is a blood thinner and purifier. It acts gently on the kidneys, and can be smelled on the urine when it is freely taken. Make a tea of it, and drink it either warm or cold at meals, instead of tea or coffee, and during the day instead of water, when you have got bad blood.

Lobelia Inflata. Lobelia. This is a very common remedy, known well to all civilization, therefore it is not necessary for me to dwell on the plant long. It is of great importance in the treatment of many diseases. It is perfectly safe for a man to administer who knows its effects. I have given it in hundreds of cases without fear, with very happy results. This remedy was discovered by a man by the name of [Samuel] Thomson. He first fully satisfied himself that it had emetic properties by coaxing his partner, who was mowing with him in the field, to chew the green plant, which he did, and became deadly sick and relaxed, and upon drinking some water he vomited and rapidly recovered from its effects, and felt better afterwards than he did before. Thomson was one of the first botanic or herb doctors, and did a great deal for suffering mankind by discovering that herbs had many valuable medical properties, that have since been used by all physicians.

Medical properties and uses. Lobelia is one of our most valuable emetics, and is only fit to be handled by a physician who knows well his business. It is one of the essentials in the croup syrup that is dealt out by many of our best doctors. I will here give you a formula:

Acetic tincture of Lobelia	one ounce.
Acetic tincture of Squill	one ounce.
Camphorated tincture of Opii	⅛ ounce.
Simple Syrup	four ounces.

Dose, a teaspoonful every two or three hours in a case of bad cold or cough. In a case of croup, every five to ten minutes, until vomiting occurs.

Stomach Bitters. Similar to Hostetter's [a well-known patent medicine].

Gentian Root, ground	½ ounce.
Cinchona Bark, ground	½ ounce.
Orange Peel, ground	½ ounce.
Cinnamon, ground	¼ ounce.
Anise Seed, ground	½ ounce.
Coriander Seed, ground	½ ounce.
Cardamom Seed, ground	⅓ ounce.
Gum Kino, ground	¼ ounce.
Alcohol	1 pint.
Water	4 quarts.
Sugar	1 pound.

Soak the drugs in the alcohol for one week, pour off the tincture, boil the drugs for a few moments in one quart of water, strain, add the tincture, the rest of the water, and sugar. Then you will have a very pleasant and mild stomach tonic and bitters that will promote digestion and guard your system against malaria or chills. Dose, a common swallow or a wine glass full before each meal and on going to bed.

Farmer's Bitters.

Tansy	¼ ounce.

Crushed Gentian Root	1 ounce.
Pulverized Hydrastis Canadensis	1 ounce.
Anise Seed	½ ounce.
Whisky	1 quart.

After standing fourteen days it is ready for use, and will be found to be a fine appetizer and a good stomach tonic, as well as a blood purifier. Dose, a common swallow three or four times a day.

German Bitters.

German Chamomile	2 ounces.
Sweet Flag	2 ounces.
Orris Root	4 ounces.
Coriander Seed	1 ½ ounce.
Centaury	1 ounce.
Orange Peel	3 ounces.
Alcohol	4 pints.
Water	4 pints.
Sugar	4 ounces.

Grind the drugs to a coarse powder, percolate with the alcohol and water, filter, and add the sugar. Dose, a tablespoonful three or four times a day.

Hop Bitters.

Hops	4 ounces.
Orange Peel	2 ounces.
Cardamom	2 drachms.
Cinnamon	1 drachm.
Cloves	½ drachm.
Alcohol	8 ounces.
Sherry Wine	2 pints.
Simple Syrup	1 pint.

Grind the drugs, macerate in the alcohol and wine for one week, percolate, add the syrup, and enough water to make one gallon. Dose, a wineglassful three or four times a day.

Stoughton Bitters.

Orange Peel, ground	6 ounces.
Gentian Root, ground	8 ounces.
Virginia Snake Root, ground	1 ½ ounce.
American Saffron, ground	½ ounce.
Red Saunders, ground	½ ounce.
Alcohol	4 pints.
Water	4 pints.

Mix, macerate fourteen days, filter, and add enough diluted alcohol to make one gallon. Dose, a tablespoonful three times a day before meals.

Corns. They are not dangerous. I never knew them to cause lockjaw or death, but yet they are equal to an aching tooth, and torment their owners severely. They are caused usually by tight shoes pressing on some part so as to check the capillary circulation and as soon as that is checked the skin becomes calloused or hardened and presses on the nerves, causing great pain. There are two kinds of corns, soft, and hard. A soft corn is found between the toes; hard ones on the outer surface. Can corns be cured? My answer is, yes, by all means. The corn may be cured in a very short time. If the patient will do as I tell him he soon can get well. Bathe the foot twice a day in hot water, and after each bathing rub with Spanish Oil or King of Pain. Wear a slipper or a loose shoe. Pare the callous to the quick just so as not to cause bleeding, and in a short time your corns will be well. Tight boots will bring them back again.

Corn Poem.

People violate nature's laws,
Which truely is disease's cause;
Tight boots they wear without a fear,
But corns you know will then appear.

Nature has the strictest way,
Who violates will get their pay,
In bunions and those cursed corns,
Which pain the feet as bad as thorns.

Thus J. I. Lighthall's Corn Extractor
Is warranted to be an actor,

And when applied upon your corn,
Removes a scale as hard as horn.

Never causing any sore,
Causing blood to run or pour.
A bottle costs you fifty cents,
Saving pain and great expense.

If people who are suffering from corns will do as I have told them, they can most certainly cure themselves and rid their feet of such miserable and tortuousome [*sic*] afflictions.

Antidote for Tobacco.

White Oak Bark, pulverized	4 ounces.
Capsicum	4 grains.

Moisten with gum arabic sufficient to make it stick together. A chew is about the size of a bean several times a day. In three or four days desire for tobacco will be gone. Whenever you want tobacco take a chew of this preparation.

How to Quit Using Opium. Commence with the same dose [of opium] in solution, and every time a dose is taken replace it with the same amount of water, and when the solution gets to be so weak that its effects are not felt, commence taking quinine in from three to five grain doses every four hours until you have taken it four or five days. Whisky and wine may be used lightly as the dose of the opiate grows smaller. The habit can be broken in four weeks, and God knows it is a fearful habit to be chained to, and no man would ever acquire it if he knew what a monster it is to overcome. The habit of getting drunk is an angel by the side of it.

Thompson's Eye Water.

Sulphate of Copper	10 grains.
Sulphate of Zinc	40 grains.
Rose Water	2 pints.
Tincture of Saffron	4 drachms.
Tincture of Camphor	4 drachms.

Mix and filter. Drop a few drops in the eyes three or four times a day.

Cough Syrup.

Tincture of Squill	2 ounces.
Tincture of Lobelia	2 ounces.

Boneset, Hops, and Hoarhound Candy.

Fluid Extract of Boneset	2 ounces.
Tincture of Hops	½ ounce.
Tincture of Blood Root	½ ounce.
Hoarhound Fluid Extract	1 ounce.
White Sugar	24 ounces.

Boil the mixture until a drop on a cold plate solidifies or gets hard. Divide while warm into little sticks, and then set it away till cool. This forms a fine candy for colds, coughs, hoarseness, minister's sore throat, and consumption.

Remedy for Burns.

Carbolic Acid	1 drachm.
Bicarbonate of Soda	1 ounce.
Linseed Oil	8 ounces.

This is the best dressing in the world for burns. It should be applied with linen or cotton batting to exclude the air from the raw surface. It should be applied as much as once or twice in twenty-four hours.

The Great Kidney Remedy. This prescription is worthy of everyone's notice who is troubled with kidney troubles, weak back, and scanty secretions of urine. Good for the horse and cow as well as man.

Tincture of Buchu	2 ounces.
Tincture of Uva Ursi	2 ounces.
Sweet Spirits of Nitre	2 ounces.
Alcohol	2 ounces.
Tincture of Juniper Berries	2 ounces.
Oil of Eucalyptus	20 drops.

Cut the oil with the two ounces of alcohol first, then mix them altogether, shaking well before taking. Dose, a teaspoonful three or four times a day until the trouble is relieved. This will be found to be by all who use it one of the finest preparations in the world. It will even cure gonorrhea. I have known this preparation to cure cases that were said by doctors to be beyond the power and reach of medicine. Whenever it acts too strong on the kidneys the dose must be lessened one-half.

To My Many Readers. I will close by saying to you, use your own judgment, uninfluenced by any prejudice that may have previously existed in your minds. Give my advice a trial if you need it, and judge me and what I say by the effects. I give you my word and honor most solemnly, that all I have told you is safe for the most delicate person to try, without the slightest danger of producing any effect detrimental, either temporary or permanent. A wise person will glean knowledge from whatever source it may arise. The compass of the Indian is the moss on the north side of the tree, which is knowledge from a natural source gleaned by the wild untutored savage. I will close by saying, good education is the only reliable means of lasting reforms, and that will teach people to think for themselves, and that simple medical facts have been hidden in the past by technical words, but today are told in common English.

Classification of Medicines, and Different Theories. I shall give you, in this essay, the names of each school of medicine, and define briefly the names of the different classifications of medicine.

Antipathy. This is a school of medicine that believes in treating diseases by giving medicine or using means that produce effects of a character that are directly opposed to the symptoms of the disease itself. They, therefore, are termed believers in what is expressed by the Latin term, "Contraria contrariis opponenda." To illustrate the idea to your minds clearly, I will say this: They claim that the first effect of opium is to constipate the bowels, or make the bowels costive, and that the second effect is diarrhea, which I know is a fact by actual experience, and by trying it on my own body. If any doctor doubts it let him try it at the peril of his life.

Homeopathy. This school was founded by Dr. Hahnemann upon the theory expressed in Latin, "Similia similibus curantur," or in English words, medicines that will produce effects like the disease in existence should be used for the cure of it. To illustrate the idea clearly I will say this: Take and burn an old dog-day sore on a boy's leg that will not heal, with lunar caustic, and immediately a healthy action will set in and the sore will heal. I will say this as a substitute for the Latin term given above: The hair of the dog is good for the bite.

Allopathy. Their method is based on the fact that their medicine will cure in a phenomenal manner, which is, I think, very near the truth. A dose of calomel will do so and so. We have an idea how it does it, or a theory fixed in our own minds, but the fact is, we are not positively certain how it does it, or what is the modus operandi. If we have an aching tooth and apply a mustard poultice on the cheek, the pain will soon stop. Now is this Homeopathy or Allopathy? Does it cure by producing an effect on the nerves causing greater pain than the toothache, or does it call the excess of circulation of blood away to the surface that is going on in the nerve of the tooth, by attracting nervous attention, or is it simply an excess of nervous attention to the pain on the outside from the mustard plaster over the pain produced by the tooth? Now, who knows for certain what the modus operandi is? An epileptic fit can be warded off by slapping the patient in the face, or by throwing cold water in the face when it first begins to come on. Often have I seen men, when they have been drinking hard, the next morning try to take a drink of whiskey, and upon swallowing it become sick, but by pinching their ears and chewing lemon or cloves, or slapping themselves in the face, would manage, by so doing, to keep it down.

Brunonian Theory. There is a theory called the Brunonian theory advocated first by a man named John Brown, M.D., who argued that all medicines acted on the human organization as stimuli or stimulants. But his theory never gained any note in the estimation of the medical world.

The twin sister to this theory is called the contra-stimulus theory, which was first believed in by Rosoria and Borda, and subsequently by other oriental doctors, but it never gained much note. The theory is too thin in its logic and reason.

The Chrono-Thermal Theory. Is simply a theory containing a few facts and many imaginative theories that are futile and worthless. I claim that there can be much knowledge gleaned, of importance and benefit to man in his practice, from this theory. Man can learn an important lesson from the ant and the bee; the lesson of industry and providing for a rainy day. So can a thinking man learn from all that is around him.

Hydropathy or Water Cure. This, so far as it goes, is a very excellent remedy. It is a complete antidote for dirtiness, when properly applied. I pronounce it a complete specific, in combination with good soap, for filthy, dirty hands, faces, and bodies. The effect, so far as it goes, results in cleanliness, which the Bible tells us is the next thing to Godliness. Man can live longer without food than he can without water. Every one knows that this fact is established beyond question or doubt by actual experiment. Water is one of the finest remedies we have in the treatment of all diseases, most especially diseases of a febrile character; but common sense teaches us that it is not a cure-all and the only remedy and the best one for the cure of diseases, free from the aid of other remedies. Never deny a sick person water when they crave it; never deny them food. Use common sense and give them what they crave.

Electicism—The Free Thinker of Medicine. The right to choose the best from all of the one idea theories of medicine; liberty uncircumscribed by the teachings of fanatics; freedom to judge for yourself that which is best of all; that you can learn of the many ideas of medical men of the world. Love for all, hatred toward none; freedom of thought; the right to counsel with all, ungoverned by a mean disgraceful code of ethics. Liberty to exercise good common sense, and use that which is best calculated to do good in the case in which it is indicated. This is the true definition of Electicism. They are the most prosperous class of doctors on the face of the world, because they believe in personal liberty as well as general liberty, and that which is right, and hate smart fanatics. [Elsewhere in his book, Lighthall refers to this group by its correct name, the Eclectics. It is curious that he alters the word here.]

Quackopathy. There is a class of doctors that are drawn from all the schools of medicine that profess to be that which they are not. They may possess diplomas, but they got them upon examination day, by some student, that had studied hard and well and was naturally sharp, helping them and cheating the professors. They never merited a diploma. They spent their time in bar rooms and at billiard tables when they should have been burning midnight oil over Gray's Anatomy, or Huxley and Dalton's Physiology, in order that they might not butcher poor suffering humanity, and have more knowledge of the human system, and know better how to prescribe medicine to those who need it, and therefore this being a fact, every one should be on their guard. It is not the man that has the diploma that is always the good doctor. I know several men that have no diplomas, that are naturally inclined in that direction, that have good success, and are men that study the human organization and the effects of medicine on it, and try to improve their moments, in order that they may properly fit themselves for usefulness, and to benefit humanity. From the fact that so many force themselves through college, a diploma does not always signify that they are fit to prescribe or issue medicine. It is the man that makes medicine a study, and studies it constantly and diligently, thinking for himself, reasoning from cause to effect, using common sense in all things, and when he or they give medicine, are sure they are right, and give it so it won't do any harm if it does no good. There are more quacks that have diplomas than there are quacks that have not. I once knew a doctor that thought himself wise, and boasted over twenty-five years experience, and when I asked him about golden seal and black cohosh, he laughed at me, and said he had never stooped so low; that they were simply granny remedies. God pity such men.

Appendix B: Handwritten Medical Formulas of George Halleck Center

Twenty-eight of George Halleck Center's recipes, covering a wide range of afflictions, are preserved on signed, handwritten (undated) cards. They are identified as follows: Tooth Powder; For Rheumatism; Center's Salve; Center's Black Root Capsules for the Liver (version no. 1); Center's Black Root Capsules for the Liver (version no. 2); Tinctures How to Make; Emetic Tincture; Liveon; Tincture of Rhubarb as used in (original) Liveon; Ozark for the Blood; Tarine Tablets (for catarrh); Center's Mouthwash and Sorethroat Gargle; Tapeworm; Center's Mother's Favorite Salve; Center's Liniment; Dyspeptic Pills; Center's Eye Balm (version no. 1); Center's Eye Balm (version no. 2); Center's Buchu Capsules for the Kidneys; Cholera Prescription; Center's Nerve Capsules; Center's Lirusan Capsules; Center's ITSPEP (for cough, colds); Center's Powdered Tar (for making Lirusan, version no. 1); Center's Powdered Tar (for making Lirusan, version no. 2); Center's Stomach Capsules; Alternative Very Strong (purgative?); Center's Extract of Wild Cheery [*sic*] for ITSPEP. Seven of the twenty-eight recipes are presented on the following pages. At least three other remedies, Liveon Liver Discs, a laxative called Mississippi Valley, and Kaskasia for rheumatism, are not represented in the extant cards.

Cholera prescription

Laudnam	2. oz.
Spirits of Camphor	2. oz.
Tincture of Ginger	1. oz.
Essence of peppermint	2. oz.
Hoffmanns anodyne	2. oz.
Or Sulphuric ether	1. oz.
Tincture of Capsicum	½. oz.

Dose. Adults 15 to 20 drops
every 20 minutes until
releived

Good for belly ache.
Shake the bottle until the
contents are well mixed.
May prevent serious trouble.

Geo H Center.

Center's
Black Root Capsules
For the liver.

Rhubarb root   4. oz.

Black root   6. oz.

Fennel Seed   2. oz.

Aloes   1. oz.

Gamboge   2. oz.

Sassafras root   1. oz.

Sulphur   2. oz.

Mix well. In a bowl.

It is now ready for use.

Dose. Adults. 1 or 2 capsules,
every hour for four hours.
Then 1 capsule every 3
hours.

For the liver.

Geo H Center.

CENTER'S ITSPEP

10 Pounds [...] brown sugar.
3 Quarts of apple vinegar
3 Quarts of extract of wild
cherry bark.
One small can of pure pine
tar.
Put all this in one vessel.
Cook slow. When it comes to
boil, let it boil for 1 hour ~~45 minutes~~
Let it cool, skim and bottle
Excellent
For colds, coughs and bronchitis
Dose. Adults one teaspoonful
morning, noon and night.
Can be taken oftener if
necessary
Geo H. Center
Locust Hill Medicine Co;
Du Quoin, Illinois.

Liveon

Tincture Rhubarb.
To Make One Pint.
Glycerine   3/4 oz.
Fluid Ext. Rhubarb 2 oz.
Fill the rest With
diluted Alcohol.

To dilute the Alcohol.
use 2 parts water to
one part alcohol.

One Pint of This
Tincture to One Gal.
of Liveon.
          Geo H. Center.

Center's

Mothers Favorite Salve

Beef Tallow	4. oz.
Bees Wax	4. oz.
Honey	4. oz.
Brown vasaline	4. oz.
Sweet Oil	4. oz.
Goose Grease	4. oz.
Rosin	4. oz.
Pure Hog Lard	1. oz.

Cook Slow. and well.
Stir while cooking.
Good for all trouble where
a salve can be used
Bath the parts with warm
water. Then use the salve

Geo H Center.

Center's
Nerve Capsules.

Yellow Lady Slipper   16 oz.
Assafetida   8 oz.
Sassafras root   2' oz
Fennel Seed   2 oz.

All in powder
Mix well. It is then
ready to put in capsules

For nervous people

Dose. Adults. 1 Capsule
every 2 or 3 hours.

Locust Hill Medicine Co.
Du Quoin, Illinois
Geo H. Center.

Tinctures How to Make.

Take 2 oz. of any
Root, Herb, Bark, Leaf
or Gum, which you
wish to use.
Bruise it. Then pour
½ pint boiling water
upon it. And when
cold add, ½ pint
Alcohol.

Keep warm for 4 or 6
days. or let stand
for 12 or 14 days it
is then ready for
use.

Geo H. Center

Contributors

Patrick Brophy is a writer on regional history and other subjects and curator of the Bushwhacker Museum in Nevada, Missouri.

Gene Fowler is a playwright, actor, and nonfiction writer. His previous books include *Border Radio* and *Crazy Water.* A resident of Austin, Texas, he has appeared professionally at the Kennedy Center, the White Elephant Saloon (Fort Worth), Contemporary Arts Museum (Houston), the San Antonio Rodeo, a Del Rio shopping mall, and on the Nashville Network.

A native of Detroit and graduate of Harvard University, Christina C. Z. Jensen writes fiction, nonfiction articles, and public relations materials from her home in Minden, Nebraska. She has worked as a ghostwriter and as a grant writer, primarily for rural hospitals. She is a board member of the Nebraska Humanities Council and teaches part time in the English Department of the University of Nebraska at Kearney.

James Marten is a Professor of History at Marquette University in Milwaukee, with a special interest in the Civil War.

Adrienne Mayor is a folklorist who publishes articles on natural history in classical antiquity and modern times. She resides in Princeton, New Jersey, and Bozeman, Montana. Michele Angel, of Minneapolis, Minnesota, is a graphic artist who maintains a deep interest in mysterious natural phenomena. As children they played (gingerly) with George Halleck Center's stuffed Gila monster, coiled snakes, and snapping turtles and were fascinated to hear about their great-grandfather's medicine wagon. They have never had their fill of stories told about Center by their grandmother Frankie, father John Mayor, great-uncle Jed, and great-aunt Ida.

Cindi Myers is a lifelong Texan who enjoys sharing the diverse history of her home state with others. Her articles have appeared in *Texas Highways, True West, Historic Traveler,* and other publications.

The late Frank Bishop Putnam was a longtime treasurer of the Historical Society of Southern California. His article on Teresa Urrea was discovered among his papers by his descendants.

Eric V. Sorg has lectured on, and performed as, Bill Cody internationally, including appearances on national television. Sorg became interested in Frank Powell after giving a program on Cody in Encampment, Wyoming, and discovering that Frank Powell and Bill Cody had owned a gold mine there. The fact that Frank Powell barely commands a dozen footnotes in Cody biographies offended Sorg, and he undertook a five-year search to uncover the real Frank Powell. Sorg received a "Publication Grant" from the Colorado Endowment for the Humanities to complete a biography on Powell, and he has published and lectured on White Beaver extensively. Sorg resides in Laramie, Wyoming.

Ferenc M. Szasz is Professor of History at the University of New Mexico in Albuquerque. Author of over seventy articles, he has also written or edited six books.

Index